THE Low Carb Cookbook
& WEIGHT LOSS PLAN

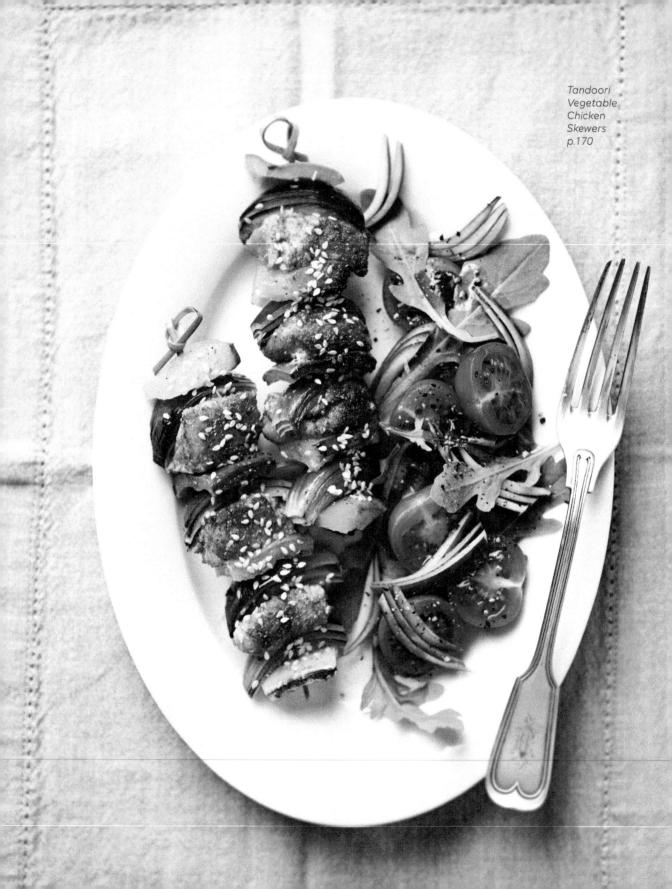

Tandoori
Vegetable
Chicken
Skewers
p.170

THE Low Carb Cookbook

& WEIGHT LOSS PLAN

21 Days to Cut Carbs & Burn Fat with a Ketogenic Diet

PAMELA ELLGEN

ROCKRIDGE
PRESS

PHOTO CREDITS: *Cover:* Tara Donne/Offset; Mint and Lemon/Shutterstock. *Back cover:* B.&.E.Dudzinski/Stockfood; Harald Walker/Stocksy; ELLIE BAYGULOV/Stocksy. *Interior:* B.&.E.Dudzinski/Stockfood, p.2; Shannon Douglas, p.6; Maya Visnyei/Stockfood, p.8; Nadine Greeff, p.12; PhotoCuisine/Kanako/Stockfood, p.22; ALIE LENGYELOVA/Stocksy, p.30; Gräfe & Unzer Verlag/Jörn Rynio/Stockfood, p.52; Great Stock!/Stockfood, p.70; ELLIE BAYGULOV/Stocksy, p. 86; Harald Walker/Stocksy, p.106; CAMERON WHITMAN/Stocksy, p.124; Gräfe & Unzer Verlag/Thorsten Suedfels/Stockfood, p.148; People Pictures/Stockfood, p.174; Leigh Beisch/Stockfood, p.200; Trent Lanz/Stocksy, p.214; The Picture Pantry/ Stockfood, p.226.

ISBN: Print 978-1-62315-928-3 | eBook 978-1-62315-929-0

To Rich,
for your love, support,
and always believing the best.

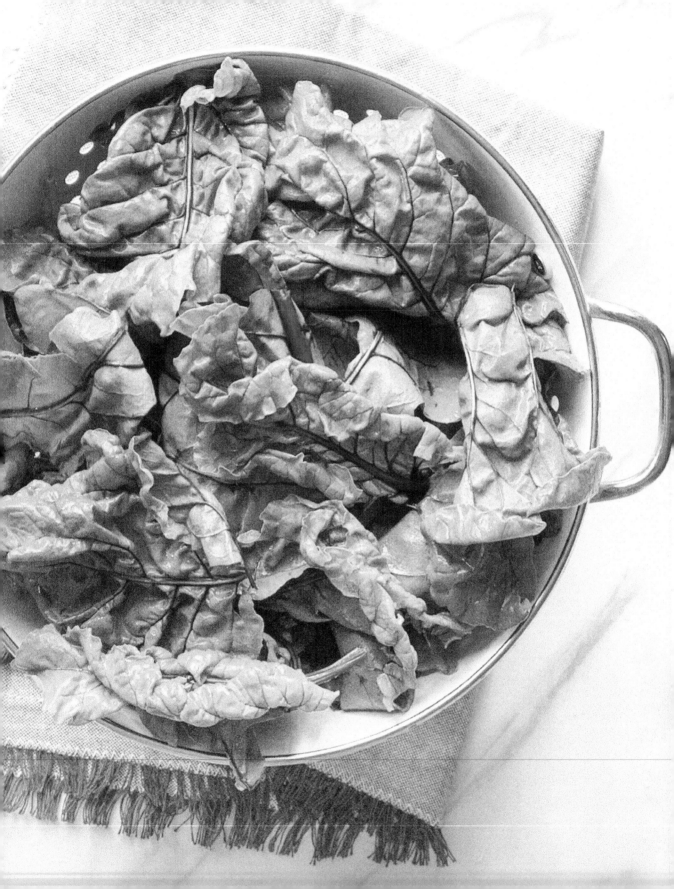

Contents

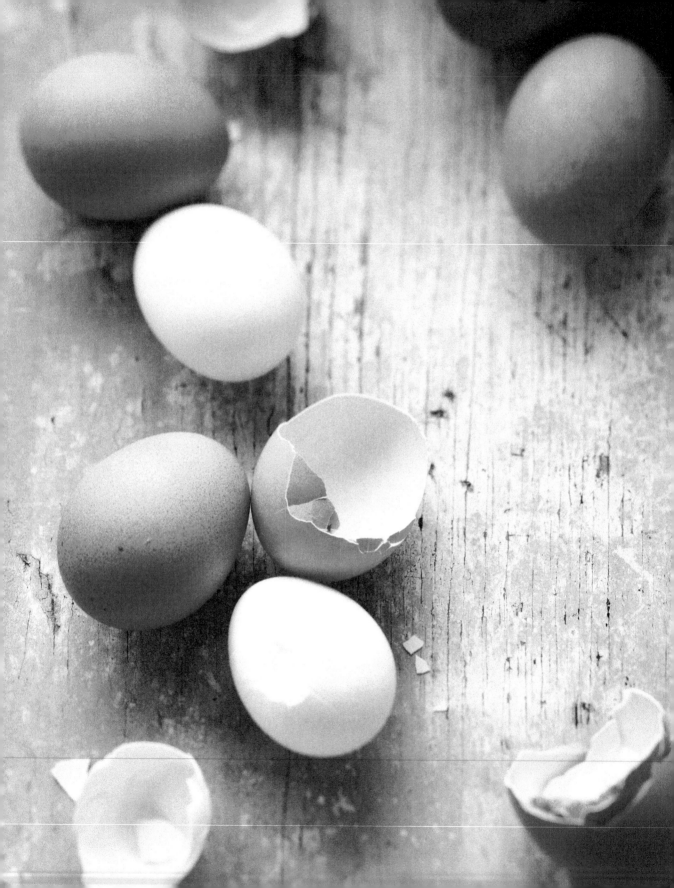

Introduction

My first attempt to lose weight involved cutting back to only one dessert a day. It was my sophomore year of college, and I had gained 20 pounds on a steady diet of pasta, pizza, fried rice, and ice cream sundaes. I ate dessert with every meal, and my favorite late-night snack was a plate of Cajun fries and ranch dressing washed down with a milkshake.

I had been a sugar addict for as long as I could remember. Growing up I could never have just a single serving of anything sweet. Once I had tasted it, I had to have more. I had no idea how addictive these foods were, and I blamed my sweet tooth and poor willpower for my insatiable desire for carbs. An active lifestyle and an otherwise healthy menu for those meals my family ate together kept me lean through my teens, but college was a different story.

Cutting back on desserts proved effective, and I lost 10 pounds over the course of a semester. The experience illustrated to me that small changes made consistently can have a profound impact and that for any diet to be successful it must be sustainable. Over the next several years, I tried many different diets to lose those last 10 pounds, but none of them provided a lasting solution. I usually felt hungry, cranky, and unhappy.

As an adult, I began to struggle with various food sensitivities and switched to a gluten-free diet, eventually adopting a low-carbohydrate, high-fat diet free from grains, legumes, dairy, and sugar and rich in fresh vegetables and fruit, meat, fish, eggs, nuts, and seeds. Instantly I saw my food cravings disappear. No longer was the plate of cookies in the office kitchen too tempting to ignore. I could go hours between meals without becoming irritable or lethargic. I finally felt like I was in control of what I ate.

And that is what I want for you.

In this book, I show you how to ditch the carbs and excess pounds without giving up flavor or feeling like you're starving. When you switch from burning glucose as your primary fuel—the natural result of a high-carb diet—to burning fat instead, you will lose weight, feel satisfied, and finally be in control of what you eat. It is such an empowering feeling!

My approach is flexible and takes into account that life happens. Unlike other diets that require you to start all over again if you deviate by even a crumb, this program rejects the all-or-nothing approach. If you exceed your carbs one day, let it go and move on to the next day. With dedication you will lose weight, change your relationship with food, and change your life!

PART ONE

The Plan

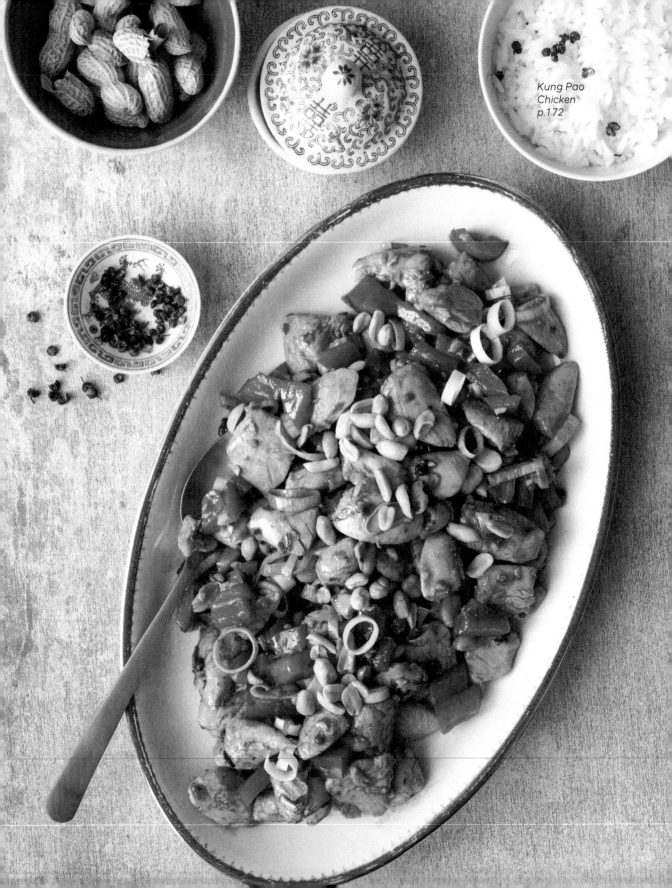

Kung Pao
Chicken
p.172

CHAPTER ONE
The Evolution of Low Carb

The low-carbohydrate diet has been around since the beginning of human history. Preagricultural humans subsisted on what they could hunt or gather, which meant wild meat, game, fish, roots, berries, and other plant matter. Around 12,000 years ago, humans left their nomadic ways and began consuming more carbohydrates in the forms of cereal grains and legumes. Still, it was a far cry from today's endless supply of pasta and breadsticks.

Fast forward to the twentieth century when industrial food products, refined grains, and sugar became widely available and came with a side of obesity, heart disease, and diabetes. Instead of blaming refined carbs—which were novel foods in human evolution—people pointed the finger at fat.

It made sense. With nine calories per gram, fat seemed like a natural enemy. Carbs and protein offered less than half that amount—only four calories per gram—so dieters loaded up on bagels, margarine, nonfat yogurt, and aspartame. Weight loss was a calories-in-calories-out equation, so high-calorie fat was out. "If it's fat free, it must be healthy," was the mantra of the day.

The only problem is that it doesn't work, at least not in the long run.

Science journalist Gary Taubes thoroughly outlines this reality in his book *Why We Get Fat: And What to Do About It*, where he writes, "The science tells us that obesity is ultimately the result of a hormonal imbalance, not a caloric one—specifically, the stimulation of insulin secretion caused by eating easily digestible, carbohydrate-rich foods. These carbohydrates literally make us fat, and by driving us to accumulate fat, they make us hungrier and they make us sedentary."

If you have ever tried dieting by restricting calories, you know the routine all too well—nagging hunger, temporary weight loss, lack of energy, and ultimately weight gain.

Fortunately, there is a better option: a low-carbohydrate, high-fat ketogenic diet. A ketogenic diet is one in which the body burns fat for fuel rather than glucose. It is grounded in decades of research and millennia of human history. It will keep you feeling full and energized while mobilizing your fat stores to fuel your everyday activity and ultimately help you lose weight. Even better, a low-carb diet is filled with all of the foods you love. Think Thai Chicken Skewers with Peanut Sauce (page 83), BBQ Baby Back Ribs (page 189), and Cream Cheese Pound Cake (page 206).

Give Up Carbs, Not Flavor

To understand why a diet low in carbohydrates is so effective, it helps to have a basic scientific understanding of how and why our bodies use and store carbohydrates.

Whenever we eat foods containing carbohydrates, our blood sugar (also known as blood glucose) levels rise proportionate to the total amount of carbohydrates we have eaten (called the glycemic load) and how quickly that carbohydrate is absorbed (called the glycemic index). The pancreas, which is an organ that's located deep in the abdomen, releases the hormone insulin, which lowers blood glucose and makes it available to the cells.

When the body doesn't need glucose for immediate energy or to restore the energy stored in the muscles (called glycogen), the glucose is repackaged with fatty acids into more complex structures called triglycerides for long-term storage within the fat cells. If there isn't enough room in the existing fat cells, new fat cells are created, aided by insulin. Insulin also activates enzymes that increase fat storage and prevent fat from being used for fuel. Hence, when blood glucose levels and insulin production remain consistently high, fat storage is inevitable and fat metabolism (that is, the use of fat for fuel) cannot occur.

A low-carbohydrate, high-fat ketogenic diet keeps insulin levels low, which allows triglycerides to be broken down into fatty acids that can be burned as energy. Not only does this result in the loss of body fat, but it also ensures that a steady stream of energy is available to fuel your body. And it tastes pretty good, too!

Have You Met These Healthy Fats?

The ketogenic diet is necessarily high in fats. But not all fats are created equal. Partially hydrogenated oils contain trans fats (even when the package says "0 grams trans fat") and are found in margarine, peanut butter, and other processed foods. They are dangerous to your health because they increase inflammation and elevate LDL ("bad" cholesterol) and reduce HDL ("good" cholesterol), both of which increase the risk of heart disease and hinder weight loss. So just go with the real stuff. Here are my top five fats for a low-carb diet:

Avocados

Avocados are rich in monounsaturated fats, particularly oleic acid, which has been shown to decrease inflammation, lower the risk of heart disease, and improve insulin sensitivity. Monounsaturated fats are burned at a faster rate than other fats and increase metabolism. For example, a study published in 2013 found that the addition of half of an avocado with meals increased satiety for up to five hours following a meal among obese individuals. Avocados are also a great source of vitamin K, folate, vitamin C, potassium, and vitamin E. Potassium is especially important on a low-carb diet because it helps prevent muscle cramping, which can be a concern as you shed excess water weight.

Butter

It is no surprise that butter contributes flavor and a rich, velvety texture to foods, but you may be surprised to learn that butter, especially when it is sourced from organic, grass-fed cows, contains omega-3 fats, selenium, and vitamins A, D, E, and K. Butter has a low smoke point, so rather than using it for high-temperature cooking, use butter on cooked vegetables, in baking, or in quick, low-heat cooking methods, such as when making eggs. If you are sensitive to dairy proteins, try ghee (also called clarified butter), which has been heated and strained to remove the milk solids.

Coconut Oil

Coconut oil is the ketogenic dieter's best friend. It is a flavorful source of fatty acids that have been shown to correlate with increased calorie burning and weight loss. It is also easily converted into water-soluble molecules called ketone bodies in the liver, meaning you can get into ketosis more quickly by adding coconut oil to your diet (see "What Is Ketosis?" opposite). Coconut oil also increases metabolism while reducing appetite, so the calories you consume from coconut oil will be burned off and cause you to eat fewer other foods. It can be eaten raw in fat bombs (sweet or savory snack bites that provide nearly all of their calories from fat) or used for roasting, sautéing, or frying.

Extra-Virgin Olive Oil

Extra-virgin olive oil is rich in monounsaturated fats, contains antioxidants, is anti-inflammatory, may reduce the risk of heart disease, and ultimately can help you lose weight. For example, a study comparing the effects of a low-fat diet versus a diet enriched with extra-virgin olive oil found that women following a 1,500-calorie-a-day diet containing three tablespoons of olive oil lost twice as much weight as those consuming the same number of calories without the olive oil. For the greatest health benefits, use extra-virgin olive oil for low-heat cooking, in salad dressings, and to drizzle over cooked foods.

Nuts

Nuts such as walnuts, cashews, pistachios, almonds, and pecans contain monounsaturated and polyunsaturated fats, including omega-3 fatty acids, and can help reduce the risk of heart disease, lower diabetes risk, and encourage you to stick with your low-carb diet by improving satiety and ultimately helping you lose weight. Nuts contain about equal proportions of protein and carbohydrate, which is mostly in the form of fiber.

WHAT IS KETOSIS?

Ketosis is a state in which your body burns fat instead of glucose for fuel. When you significantly reduce carbohydrates in your diet, your liver produces molecules called ketones from stored body fat, which can be used for energy. This process is natural, and your body is in a light state of ketosis when you wake up in the morning, before you eat breakfast.

"Fat adaptation" is another term that describes ketosis. Being in ketosis naturally reduces your appetite. In fact, appetite reduction is one of the many appeals of fat adaptation because you can go for long stretches between meals—such as a busy day or a deliberate period of fasting—without feeling hungry or experiencing symptoms of low blood sugar.

In healthy people, nutritional ketosis is usually achieved within as few as three days of reducing daily carbohydrate intake to below 50 grams. However, people who are obese may have more difficulty achieving ketosis. Ketosis can also be induced by fasting, which counterintuitively may be easier for some people than eating a low-carb diet during the transition period. Always consult your physician before making any dietary changes.

A ketogenic diet may improve metabolic syndrome, insulin resistance, and type 2 diabetes. It is also used to treat people with epilepsy and other neurological disorders.

Going Keto

A ketogenic diet contains low carbohydrates, moderate protein, and high fat. The macronutrient composition of a ketogenic diet typically falls within the following ranges: 5 to 10 percent carbohydrates, 20 to 25 percent protein, and 70 percent fat. On a 2,000-calorie-per-day diet, that would look like 50 grams of carbohydrates, 100 grams of protein, and 155 grams of fat.

Some low-carbohydrate diets include very high levels of protein—as high as 50 percent of total calories. While protein promotes satiety, improves mood, and builds muscle, obtaining more than 30 percent of your calories from protein can have detrimental and even dangerous effects. Excess protein can be converted to glucose, which elevates insulin levels, hinders ketosis, and may stall weight loss. Worse yet, excess protein can cause kidney damage, weaken bones, and contribute to the growth of cancer cells.

Instead of replacing calories from carbohydrates with calories from protein, the ketogenic approach involves replacing those calories with calories from fat. Pairing a low-carbohydrate diet with a high-fat diet is essential to success because even during weight loss, your body can only burn a limited amount of stored body fat—about 69 calories per kilogram of nonessential body fat per day. You have to eat something to fuel your daily activity, and dietary fat is the best replacement for carbs. Dietary fat slows the release of glucose into the bloodstream and is satiating, so you won't feel hungry on a low-carb diet. Of course, always speak to your doctor before beginning any diet, especially if you have an existing medical condition.

Should You Count Calories?

While calories do matter even on a ketogenic diet, they don't *necessarily* need to be counted because ketosis results in a natural appetite reduction and reduced calorie intake. Nevertheless, calculating your basal metabolic rate (BMR) and total daily energy expenditure (TDEE) is useful for planning purposes and can be essential if you find that your weight loss has stalled on a low-carb diet. Here's how to calculate how many calories per day you should consume for weight loss:

CALCULATE BMR

For women:	For men:
655.1 + (4.35 × ___ weight in pounds)	66 + (6.2 × ___ weight in pounds)
+ (4.7 × ___ height in inches)	+ (12.7 × ___ height in inches)
– (4.7 × ___ age in years)	– (6.76 × ___ age in years)
= Basal Metabolic Rate, BMR	= Basal Metabolic Rate, BMR

FACTOR IN ACTIVITY

Multiply your BMR by your activity level to determine your TDEE.

- Sedentary to light exercise (1 hour per week): 1.10

- Moderate exercise (2 to 3 hours per week): 1.20

- Intense exercise (4 or more hours per week): 1.35

BMR x activity level = TDEE in calories

SUBTRACT CALORIES

Subtract 20 percent from your TDEE to determine the number of calories you should consume each day. The formula is: TDEE × 0.8 = daily calories for weight loss.

If Tina weighs 190 pounds, is five feet five inches tall (65 inches), is 43 years old, and engages in moderate exercise, her BMR would be 1,586, her TDEE would be 1,903, and the number of calories she should eat daily to lose weight would be 1,522.

Measuring Ketones

To determine whether you are in ketosis, you can measure the level of ketone bodies present in your blood, breath, or urine with simple monitoring devices or pH strips. Ketone levels can be tested in the morning on an empty stomach or before bedtime. The specific ketone bodies being measured are acetoacetate, 2-hydroxybutyric acid, and acetone.

Optimal ketosis for weight loss is often defined as at least 0.5 millimoles per litre (mmol/L), but every person responds differently to a ketogenic diet. Luis Villasenor, founder of Ketogains.com, advises: "Don't chase ketones; chase results." I tend to agree with this approach.

TRANSITION TIPS

Any dietary change can be difficult to adopt, but the shift to a ketogenic diet can come with some unpleasant side effects. Here are a few strategies for easing your transition:

INCREASE ELECTROLYTES Side effects of low-carb diets may include headaches, muscle cramps, and fatigue. These are due in part to a change in electrolyte balance. When you reduce carbohydrates in your diet, your body releases stored water weight. This is fun to watch on the scale, but it isn't always pleasant to experience. Maintain adequate sodium, potassium, and other vitamin and mineral levels by drinking Bone Broth (pages 224 and 225), salting your food generously, and considering an electrolyte supplement.

TAKE IT EASY For many people the transition into ketosis can yield better sleep and plenty of energy. For others it can result in insomnia and lethargy. During the first two weeks of a low-carb diet, give yourself plenty of time to rest and plan the transition for a time when you don't have strenuous or stressful events. Also, athletic performance may suffer initially, so skip that half-marathon until after you're fully in ketosis and can reap the benefits of fat adaptation.

EAT MORE FIBER A low-carb diet may improve your digestion—especially if your diet was filled with processed foods before—but it also may slow things down and result in constipation. Vegetables contain carbohydrates, but much of them are indigestible in the form of fiber, which can improve bowel function. Aim for around 10 grams of fiber a day from vegetables.

TAKE A BREATH MINT The ketone acetone is excreted in your urine and breath and may cause your breath to smell fruity or downright stinky. Brush your teeth and floss regularly, pop a sugarless breath mint, drink plenty of water, and chew sugarless gum if you need to.

Five Steps for Weight Loss

1. **GET A PLAN.** Research indicates that dieters who have specific, measurable goals and a concrete plan to achieve them are more successful than those without them. Use the 21-day program outlined in chapter 3 as your starting point.

2. **DITCH YOUR OLD HABITS.** If you've built your life around a morning trip to the snack machine or a nightly bowl of ice cream, it's time to ditch those old habits and replace them with new routines. While you may be able to find a low-carb alternative, a better option is to replace old habits entirely with healthy, new choices. They'll feel awkward initially, but eventually they'll become your new normal.

3. **EAT LOW-CARB, HIGH-FAT.** This step should be obvious by now. Use the recipes in this book to enjoy delicious, low-carb, high-fat meals to help you enter ketosis and lose weight.

4. **BURN FAT THROUGH EXERCISE.** Although exercise isn't essential for weight loss on a low-carb diet, it is good for your mind and body. If you're new to exercise, a gentle walk is a great place to start. If you're already fit and active, keep it up. Steady-state cardio (such as light jogging, which keeps your heart rate in a moderate zone), weight training, and short bursts of high-intensity interval training have beneficial effects on your metabolism.

5. **STICK TO THE PLAN.** Three weeks is enough time to see some results, but lasting changes come from lasting choices. Continue enjoying the recipes in this book after the 21 days are over and find other cookbooks and food blogs to support your low-carb, high-fat lifestyle.

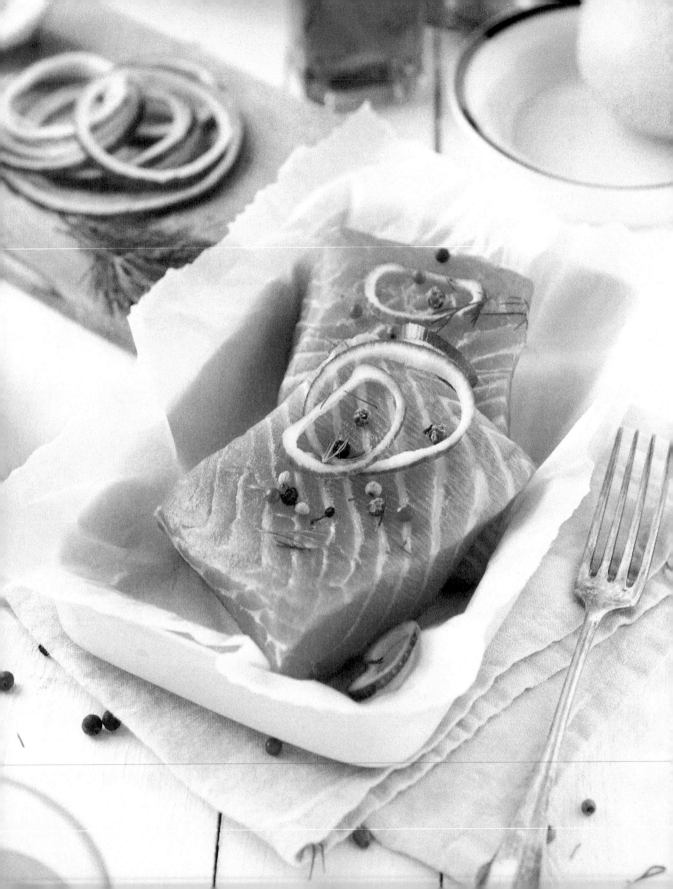

CHAPTER TWO

The Low-Carb High-Fat Kitchen

This chapter introduces you to the low-carb, high-fat kitchen and suggests pantry staples to have on hand as well as those ingredients you should probably get rid of before you start this plan. It includes how to replace high-carb foods with flavorful alternatives and tips on how to dine out successfully.

Start Fresh

Changing your diet is challenging enough, but keeping forbidden foods around the house is a recipe for frustration. Instead, purge the carb-laden foods from your refrigerator and pantry before you begin a ketogenic diet. Here are some of the most obvious offenders:

- Bread
- Cakes
- Chips
- Cookies
- Crackers
- Cupcakes
- Legumes
- Pasta
- Potatoes
- Rice
- Snack cakes
- Sweetened beverages
- Sweetened condiments and dressings
- Syrup and other sweeteners, including honey

Stock Your Refrigerator and Pantry

Clearing forbidden foods from your pantry will make it easier to stick to the plan, and you'll have that much more room for the tasty, low-carb foods you will soon be enjoying. You'll find complete shopping lists in chapter 3, but to give you an idea, here are some of the most common ingredients found in the recipes in this book:

- Bacon
- Black pepper
- Butter
- Cheese (such as cheddar, Parmesan, and mozzarella)
- Coconut oil
- Cumin
- Eggs
- Extra-virgin olive oil
- Garlic
- Ginger
- Greek yogurt, whole-milk plain
- Herbs, fresh (such as basil, cilantro, and parsley)
- Nuts
- Onions
- Paprika, smoked
- Sea salt
- Stevia, liquid
- Vinegar

Your Go-To Foods

Keeping the list of common ingredients in mind, let's now take a look at why certain staples of a low-carb diet are so essential:

LEAFY GREENS provide fiber, vitamins, minerals, antioxidants, and other micronutrients. They add volume to a low-carb diet and are both beautiful and delicious. Options include kale, chard, collard greens, arugula, romaine lettuce, and spinach, among a myriad of other delicious options.

COLORFUL non-starchy vegetables are also a pretty and tasty source of fiber and micronutrients. Options are almost endless and include asparagus, broccoli, cauliflower, endive, fennel, mushrooms, onion, peppers, radishes, and spinach. Avocado, tomato, and zucchini also fall into this category though they are technically fruits.

EGGS are one of the easiest ketogenic breakfast options. When cooked with butter, they hit the exact keto ratio of 70 percent or more fat and contain no carbs. Ideally choose free-range, organic eggs for the best nutrition and environmental sustainability.

COCONUT OIL can help suppress appetite and increase your metabolism. Choose extra-virgin, cold-pressed coconut oil for the best nutrition. If you don't like the coconut flavor, choose a filtered coconut oil. Add coconut oil into your diet slowly to avoid digestive discomfort.

CHICKEN THIGHS have so much more flavor than chicken breasts and withstand longer cooking times, especially if they are bone-in. Choose free-range, organic chicken if possible and opt for skin-on, bone-in meat. Even better, purchase a whole chicken and use the bones to make Chicken Bone Broth (page 224).

BEEF is off-limits in many modern diets, but it's a staple in most ketogenic diets. The most common cuts in low-carb diets include short ribs, ground beef, and rib eye steak. Choose grass-fed beef for the best nutrition.

BACON needs no explanation, but just in case you need convincing, bacon adds flavor, fat, and a moderate amount of protein. Choose a nitrite-free, uncured bacon for the best nutrition. My favorite is applewood smoked bacon.

FATTY FISH such as salmon, tuna, and mackerel are rich in omega-3 fatty acids and are considered heart-healthy choices. Choose wild fish whenever possible and explore sustainable options through Monterey Bay Aquarium's Seafood Watch program (SeafoodWatch.org).

BUTTER is a staple of low-carb diets, but not in the quantities you might imagine. A little goes a long way toward shifting the calorie balance to fat instead of carbs. It is especially helpful to ensure you get enough calories without overdoing it on protein. Choose butter from grass-fed cows if possible.

NUTS make great snacks and are rich in fiber and micronutrients. They also provide the crunch factor that's often lacking in low-carb diets. Choose whole nuts and weigh or measure them to ensure you're getting a proper portion. The best options are Brazil nuts, cashews, macadamia nuts, pecans, pine nuts, pistachios, and walnuts.

NO ARTIFICIAL SWEETENERS

Artificial sweeteners such as aspartame and saccharin are positively correlated with metabolic syndrome, weight gain, headaches, and even cancer. Part of the reason for their effects on weight is that they stimulate insulin production in much the same way that sugar does. Also, they train your taste buds to prefer sweet foods. Sugar alcohols are similarly problematic and often result in severe gastrointestinal distress due to their inability to be absorbed by the body.

Stevia, on the other hand, is a natural sweetener that contributes no calories or carbohydrates. However, many people with certain pollen allergies may be sensitive to stevia, so use caution when trying it for the first time. I use it sparingly in cooking, particularly for making low-carb desserts. I also use the sweetener Swerve in some baked goods. It can be used cup-for-cup to replace sugar in most recipes. It is made from erythritol, a sugar alcohol that is easier to digest than most, and which has no bitter aftertaste.

How to Reduce Carbs and Increase Flavor

You never really realize how many carbs some of your favorite foods contain until you turn over the package and start reading the nutrition label. You already know to avoid bread, potatoes, rice, and sweets on a low-carb diet, but carbs are also lurking in unlikely places. Here are some foods to limit or avoid on a low-carb diet:

5 Surprising Sources of Carbs

1. **CONDIMENTS:** Barbecue sauce and ketchup are filled with so much sugar that you might not be able to distinguish their nutrition facts from those of cake frosting, packing in 5 to 7 grams of sugar per tablespoon! Most prepared salad dressings contain added sugar, especially if they're reduced fat. Instead, create your own sauces and salad dressings using oil, vinegar, vegetables, herbs, and spices, as described in some of the recipes that follow.

2. **DAIRY:** One cup of milk contains 12 grams of carbohydrates, as many as a slice of wheat bread. Yogurt can be even worse, with as many as 19 grams of carbohydrates in a cup of plain yogurt and more than twice that in the sweetened varieties. Whole-milk (or full-fat) Greek yogurt is a better option, with 9 grams of carbs per cup. Cheese and butter are the lowest-carb dairy options, with 2 grams or fewer per cup.

3. **PEANUT BUTTER AND NUT BUTTER:** Just two tablespoons (about one ounce) of peanut butter or almond butter contain 7 grams of carbohydrates. If you're scooping it into smoothies or slathering it on low-carb bread, beware—the carbs and calories add up quickly! Only use the amounts specified in the recipes. Otherwise, whole nuts are a better option. Macadamia nuts, walnuts, and pecans all have fewer than 4 grams of carbs per ounce.

4. **PROTEIN BARS:** Processed protein supplements such as bars and powders can contain more than 20 grams of carbs per serving depending on the brand. Instead of these convenience foods, choose whole-food sources of protein such as fish, meat, eggs, nuts, and seeds, or select protein powder that is sweetened with stevia.

5. **SUGAR-FREE FOODS:** Even sugar-free foods such as pudding, jams, and cookies are often still loaded with carbs. Sugar-free jam has 5 grams of carbs per tablespoon and sugar-free pudding has 12 grams per half-cup serving. That's not to mention the artificial sweeteners, preservatives, and other chemicals these foods contain.

Ready for some good news? Some of the most flavorful foods and cooking techniques add virtually no carbs and make your ketogenic meals taste really good! And it goes without saying that just adding butter makes everything taste better. Here are my top five tips for boosting flavor on a low-carb diet:

5 Tips for Adding Flavor

1. **ADD VINEGAR:** Vinegars such as balsamic, red wine, white wine, and sherry all brighten the flavors of virtually any dish without adding carbs. I like to add a splash of vinegar near the end of the cooking period and adjust to taste. Cooking with a splash of red or white wine also boosts flavor. The alcohol cooks off in just a few minutes, leaving no carbs and a complex flavor.

2. **COOK WITH BROTH:** Use Chicken Bone Broth (page 224) or Beef Bone Broth (page 225) to braise meat, cook vegetables, stir into sauces, and of course as a base for soup.

3. **ROAST VEGETABLES:** Steaming vegetables preserves more nutrients, but roasted vegetables have an unbeatable flavor. Cook them with a generous amount of fat on a baking sheet in a hot oven for the best results.

4. **SEAR MEAT:** Cook meat briefly over high heat with a bit of fat to produce a golden-brown crust. Do this for quick-cooking steaks and chicken or tougher cuts of meat before adding wine or broth for a long, slow simmer.

5. **USE FRESH HERBS:** While dried herbs boast a long shelf life, they don't compare to fresh when it comes to flavor. Woody herbs such as thyme and rosemary can withstand long cooking periods. More delicate herbs such as cilantro, dill, and basil should be added near the end of the cooking time to get the most flavor.

About the Recipes

The recipes in this book are designed to give you 50 grams or fewer of carbohydrates each day, about 15 or fewer grams per recipe with a daily macro breakdown of 70 percent fat, 20 to 25 percent protein, and 5 to 10 percent carbohydrates. Each serving provides up to 500 calories for meals and 200 calories for side dishes, snacks, and desserts. Almost all of the recipes are naturally gluten-free. Many also fit within the Paleo diet and contain no refined vegetable oils, dairy, grains, or legumes.

The Keto Quotient at the top of each recipe refers to the percentage of fat a recipe contains—the higher the Keto Quotient, the higher the percentage of fat. Recipes with a Keto Quotient 1 have up to 69 percent of calories from fat, Keto Quotient 2 is 70 to 79 percent, and Keto Quotient 3 is 80 percent or more.

The recipes are organized with smoothies and breakfasts first, followed by snacks and starters, soups and salads, and veggies and other side dishes. The next chapters are main dishes, which are organized by protein: fish and seafood; chicken; and beef, lamb, and pork. Then, as a treat for your taste buds, there's also a chapter offering a few low-carb sweets. The recipe chapters wrap up with low-carb staples such as bone broths and sauces.

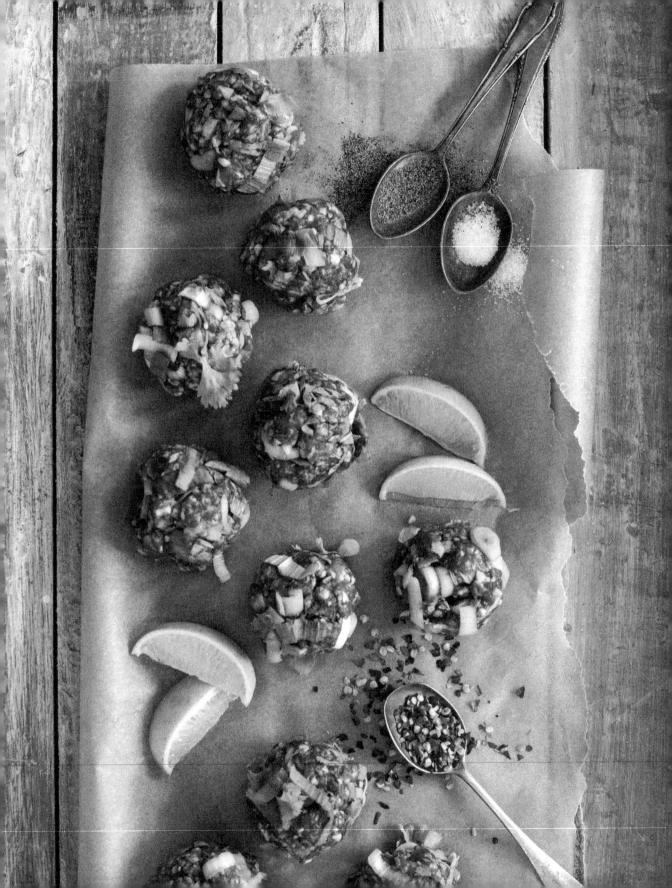

CHAPTER THREE

The First 21 Days

If you like a concrete plan with every meal outlined, this chapter is for you. It includes weekly menus, shopping lists, and daily macronutrient calculations. It also has themes for each week and motivation to help you succeed.

Each day's meals are designed to provide roughly 1,500 to 1,600 calories. In chapter 1, you calculated your total daily energy expenditure (TDEE) and the calories you need for weight loss. Use those numbers and adjust the meal plan accordingly. For example, if you should be consuming more than 1,600 calories per day, eat an additional portion at dinner or add a snack to your daily meal plan. If you need fewer calories, you can omit snacks or eat a half portion of one or more meals.

The lunch and dinner recipes in this book and on the meal plan yield four servings. The shopping list is written assuming that you will eat one portion at that meal, and, in most cases, enjoy a second portion later in the week (you will see it listed in the menu). The remaining two portions can be shared with family or friends or frozen to enjoy later.

You do not have to follow this meal plan exactly to see results. The best plan is the one that works for you. If you don't like a certain type of food, swap the recipe for another with similar nutrition values. If you don't feel like cooking every meal from scratch, just choose a handful of recipes, batch cook them at the beginning of the week, and eat a similar menu every day.

Meal Plan—Week 1

Welcome to your first week on a low-carb, ketogenic diet. This week is all about enjoying delicious foods. Dinners you will enjoy this week include Essential New York Strip Steak (page 179) with Caramelized Fennel (page 122) and Carne Asada Chicken Bowls (page 158) with a dessert of Chocolate Mousse (page 207).

Hunger is a potential pitfall when following a low-carb diet because it can often lead you down the path of temptation straight to the vending machine! To combat possible hunger or cravings, two fat bombs are introduced this week, one sweet and one savory. Also, the recipes will yield plenty of leftovers that you can snack on as needed whenever hunger strikes.

Many of the recipes in this book call for fresh herbs, such as cilantro and parsley. You can keep these herbs from wilting by storing them upright in a glass of water, covered by a plastic bag in the refrigerator. And, if possible, a windowsill herb garden would make a great addition to your low-carb kitchen.

Monday

BREAKFAST: Nutty Chocolate Protein Shake (page 54)
Calories: 368; Fat: 22g; Protein: 39g; Total Carbs: 12g; Fiber: 6g; Net Carbs: 6g
54% fat, 41% protein, 5% carbs

LUNCH: Spinach Salad with Bacon and Soft-Boiled Eggs (page 94)
Calories: 352; Fat: 30g; Protein: 16g; Total Carbs: 4g; Fiber: 2g; Net Carbs: 2g
78% fat, 18% protein, 4% carbs

SNACK: Sun-Dried Tomato and Feta Fat Bombs (page 78)
Calories: 154; Fat: 15g; Protein: 4g; Total Carbs: 3g; Fiber: 1g; Net Carbs: 2g
88% fat, 10% protein, 2% carbs

DINNER: Carne Asada Chicken Bowls (page 158)
Calories: 422; Fat: 31g; Protein: 28g; Total Carbs: 9g; Fiber: 5g; Net Carbs: 4g
66% fat, 27% protein, 7% carbs

DESSERT: Chocolate Mousse (page 207)
Calories: 288; Fat: 26g; Protein: 9g; Total Carbs: 6g; Fiber: 1g; Net Carbs: 5g
81% fat, 12% protein, 7% carbs

MONDAY'S TOTAL NUTRITION
Calories: 1,584; Fat: 124g; Protein 96g; Total Carbs: 34g; Fiber: 15g; Net Carbs: 19g
70% fat, 24% protein, 6% carbs

Tuesday

BREAKFAST: Ham and Cheese Egg Scramble (page 64)
Calories: 546; Fat: 47g; Protein: 25g; Total Carbs: 11g; Fiber: 6g; Net Carbs: 5g
77% fat, 18% protein, 5% carbs

LUNCH: Greek Salad with Shrimp (page 96)
Calories: 382; Fat: 25g; Protein: 30g; Total Carbs: 9g; Fiber: 3g; Net Carbs: 6g
59% fat, 31% protein, 10% carbs

SNACK: Peanut Butter Cookie Dough Fat Bombs (page 76)
Calories: 215; Fat: 21g; Protein: 4g; Total Carbs: 3g; Fiber: 1g; Net Carbs: 2g
88% fat, 7% protein, 5% carbs

DINNER: Essential New York Strip Steak (page 179)
Calories: 473; Fat: 36g; Protein: 38g; Total Carbs: 1g; Fiber: 0g; Net Carbs: 1g
68% fat, 32% protein, <1% carbs

TUESDAY'S TOTAL NUTRITION
Calories: 1,616; Fat: 129g; Protein: 97g; Total Carbs: 24g; Fiber: 10g; Net Carbs: 14g
71% fat, 23% protein, 6% carbs

Wednesday

BREAKFAST: Breakfast Pizza (page 69)
Calories: 431; Fat: 32g; Protein: 27g; Total Carbs: 8g; Fiber: 2g; Net Carbs: 6g
67% fat, 25% protein, 8% carbs

LUNCH: Spinach Salad with Bacon and Soft-Boiled Eggs (page 94)
Calories: 352; Fat: 30g; Protein: 16g; Total Carbs: 4g; Fiber: 2g; Net Carbs: 2g
78% fat, 18% protein, 4% carbs

DINNER: Carne Asada Chicken Bowls (page 158)
Calories: 422; Fat: 31g; Protein: 28g; Total Carbs: 9g; Fiber: 5g; Net Carbs: 4g
66% fat, 27% protein, 7% carbs

DESSERT: Chocolate Mousse (page 207)
Calories: 288; Fat: 26g; Protein: 9g; Total Carbs: 6g; Fiber: 1g; Net Carbs: 5g
81% fat, 12% protein, 7% carbs

WEDNESDAY'S TOTAL NUTRITION
Calories: 1,493; Fat: 119g; Protein: 80g; Total Carbs: 27g; Fiber: 10g; Net Carbs: 17g
72% fat, 21% protein, 7% carbs

Thursday

BREAKFAST: Nutty Chocolate Protein Shake (page 54)
Calories: 368; Fat: 22g; Protein: 39g; Total Carbs: 12g; Fiber: 6g; Net Carbs: 6g
54% fat, 41% protein, 5% carbs

LUNCH: Greek Salad with Shrimp (page 96)
Calories: 382; Fat: 25g; Protein: 30g; Total Carbs: 9g; Fiber: 3g; Net Carbs: 6g
59% fat, 31% protein, 10% carbs

SNACK: Peanut Butter Cookie Dough Fat Bombs (page 76)
Calories: 215; Fat: 21g; Protein: 4g; Total Carbs: 3g; Fiber: 1g; Net Carbs: 2g
88% fat, 7% protein, 5% carbs

DINNER: Essential Roasted Chicken (page 150)
Calories: 490; Fat: 30g; Protein: 51g; Total Carbs: 0g; Fiber: 0g; Net Carbs: 0g
55% fat, 45% protein, 0% carbs

DINNER SIDE DISH: Smoky Stewed Kale (page 117)
Calories: 190; Fat: 15g; Protein: 5g; Total Carbs: 14g; Fiber: 5g; Net Carbs: 9g
71% fat, 11% protein, 18% carbs

THURSDAY'S TOTAL NUTRITION
Calories: 1,645; Fat: 113g; Protein: 129g; Total Carbs: 38g; Fiber: 15g; Net Carbs: 23g
62% fat, 31% protein, 9% carbs

Friday

BREAKFAST: Breakfast Pizza (page 69)

Calories: 431; Fat: 32g; Protein: 27g; Total Carbs: 8g; Fiber: 2g; Net Carbs: 6g
67% fat, 25% protein, 8% carbs

LUNCH: Essential Roasted Chicken (page 150)

Calories: 490; Fat: 30g; Protein: 51g; Total Carbs: 0g; Fiber: 0g; Net Carbs: 0g
55% fat, 45% protein, 0% carbs

LUNCH SIDE DISH: Smoky Stewed Kale (page 117)

Calories: 190; Fat: 15g; Protein: 5g; Total Carbs: 14g; Fiber: 5g; Net Carbs: 9g
71% fat, 11% protein, 18% carbs

DINNER: Pan-Seared Butter Scallops (page 126)

Calories: 324; Fat: 21g; Protein: 29g; Total Carbs: 5g; Fiber: 1g; Net Carbs: 4g
59% fat, 36% protein, 5% carbs

DINNER SIDE DISH: Sautéed Zucchini with Mint and Pine Nuts (page 123)

Calories: 125; Fat: 11g; Protein: 2g; Total Carbs: 6g; Fiber: 2g; Net Carbs: 4g
79% fat, 6% protein, 15% carbs

FRIDAY'S TOTAL NUTRITION

Calories: 1,560; Fat: 109g; Protein: 114g; Total Carbs: 33g; Fiber: 10g; Net Carbs: 23g
63% fat, 29% protein, 8% carbs

Saturday

BREAKFAST: Ham and Cheese Egg Scramble (page 64)

Calories: 546; Fat: 47g; Protein: 25g; Total Carbs: 11g; Fiber: 6g; Net Carbs: 5g
77% fat, 18% protein, 5% carbs

LUNCH: Tomato Basil Chicken Zoodle Bowls (page 156)

Calories: 456; Fat: 31g; Protein: 37g; Total Carbs: 6g; Fiber: 1g; Net Carbs: 5g
61% fat, 32% protein, 7% carbs

DINNER: Slow Cooker Pork Chile Verde (page 104)

Calories: 496; Fat: 37g; Protein: 29g; Total Carbs: 11g; Fiber: 3g; Net Carbs: 8g
67% fat, 23% protein, 10% carbs

SATURDAY'S TOTAL NUTRITION

Calories: 1,498; Fat: 115g; Protein: 91g; Total Carbs: 28g; Fiber: 10g; Net Carbs: 18g
69% fat, 24% protein, 7% carbs

Sunday

BREAKFAST: Loaded Denver Omelet (page 67)
Calories: 415; Fat: 33g; Protein: 26g; Total Carbs: 4g; Fiber: 0g; Net Carbs: 4g
72% fat, 25% protein, 3% carbs

LUNCH: Slow Cooker Pork Chile Verde (page 104)
Calories: 496; Fat: 37g; Protein: 29g; Total Carbs: 11g; Fiber: 3g; Net Carbs: 8g
67% fat, 23% protein, 10% carbs

DINNER: Essential New York Strip Steak (page 179)
Calories: 473; Fat: 36g; Protein: 38g; Total Carbs: 1g; Fiber: 0g; Net Carbs: 1g
68% fat, 32% protein, <1% carbs

DINNER SIDE DISH: Caramelized Fennel (page 122)
Calories: 156; Fat: 14g; Protein: 2g; Total Carbs: 9g; Fiber: 4g; Net Carbs: 5g
79% fat, 1% protein, 20% carbs

SUNDAY'S TOTAL NUTRITION
Calories: 1,540; Fat: 120g; Protein: 95g; Total Carbs: 25g; Fiber: 7g; Net Carbs: 18g
70% fat, 25% protein, 5% carbs

Week 1 Shopping List

Canned and Bottled Items

- Almond milk, unsweetened
- Chicken broth, low-sodium (1 quart plus 4 ounces)
- Peanut butter, natural (1 small jar)
- Roasted red bell peppers (8-ounce jar)
- Salsa verde, fire-roasted (16-ounce jar)
- Sun-dried tomatoes, not oil packed (1 package)
- Tomato paste (6-ounce can)

Dairy and Eggs

- Butter (12 ounces)
- Cheddar cheese, shredded (1 small package)
- Cream cheese, full-fat (4 ounces)
- Eggs (2 dozen)
- Feta cheese (6 ounces)
- Half-and-half (1 small container)
- Heavy cream (1 small container)
- Mozzarella cheese, fresh (16 ounces)
- Pepper Jack cheese, shredded (1 small package)
- Sour cream, full-fat (1 small container)

Meat

- Bacon, applewood smoked (5 ounces)
- Chicken thighs, boneless, skinless (2 pounds)
- Chicken, whole (3 to 4 pounds)
- Ham (2 ounces)
- Italian sausage (4 ounces)
- Pork shoulder (1 pound)
- Scallops, large (1 pound)
- Shrimp, cooked (1 pound)
- Steak, New York strip (four 6-ounce steaks)

Pantry Staples

- Almond flour
- Black peppercorns
- Canola oil
- Cayenne pepper
- Chocolate, dark 85 percent cacao
- Coconut oil
- Cumin, ground
- Extra-virgin olive oil
- Pine nuts
- Protein powder, chocolate
- Red pepper flakes
- Red wine vinegar
- Sea salt
- Smoked paprika, ground
- Soy sauce, low-sodium
- Stevia, liquid
- Vanilla extract
- White wine vinegar

Produce

- Avocados (3 medium)
- Basil, fresh (1 bunch)
- Bell pepper, red (1)
- Cauliflower (1 small head)
- Cilantro, fresh (1 bunch)
- Cucumber (1 small)
- Garlic (2 heads)
- Kale (2 bunches)
- Lemon (1)
- Lettuce, romaine (2 heads)
- Lime (1)
- Mint, fresh (1 bunch)
- Onion, red (1 small)
- Onions, yellow (2 medium)
- Oregano, fresh (1 bunch)
- Parsley, fresh (1 bunch)
- Radishes (1 small bunch)
- Rosemary, fresh (1 bunch)
- Scallions (2 bunches)
- Shallots (2)
- Spinach, fresh (10 ounces)
- Tomatoes, grape (1 pint)
- Tomatoes, plum (8)
- Thyme, fresh (1 bunch)
- Zucchini (4 medium)

Meal Plan—Week 2

Congratulations, you made it through the first week on a low-carb diet and are probably seeing the numbers on the scale dropping! Some of the side effects of starting a ketogenic diet (the "keto flu") may be in full swing right now, but you've got this! The good news is that you may already be in ketosis by this week.

The theme for this week is consistency. Ultimately, for any diet to be successful, it must be sustainable. So keep up the good work and enjoy a menu that includes Slow Cooker Pork Carnitas (page 186), No-Bake Coconut Chocolate Squares (page 203), and Pepper-Crusted Salmon with Wilted Kale (page 133).

One pitfall to watch out for this week is failing to plan ahead. Try to do prep work on Sunday for the week ahead so meal preparation is a breeze during the week. You can also let the slow cooker do the work for you. Be sure to freeze extra portions to enjoy later without all the prep work.

If you're following all three weeks, you likely have many of the ingredients needed for this week's menu left over from last week, especially fresh herbs, eggs, cream cheese, butter, ham, and almond flour. Check your pantry and refrigerator before you head out to the grocery store.

Monday

BREAKFAST: Broccoli Bacon Egg Muffin Cups (page 66)
Calories: 338; Fat: 22g; Protein: 29g; Total Carbs: 4g; Fiber: 1g; Net Carbs: 3g
62% fat, 34% protein, 4% carbs

LUNCH: Curried Chicken Salad (page 154)
Calories: 379; Fat: 28g; Protein: 27g; Total Carbs: 4g; Fiber: 1g; Net Carbs: 3g
67% fat, 29% protein, 4% carbs

SNACK/DESSERT: No-Bake Coconut Chocolate Squares (page 203)
Calories: 144; Fat: 16g; Protein: 1g; Total Carbs: 2g; Fiber: 1g; Net Carbs: 1g
98% fat, 1% protein, 1% carbs

DINNER: Slow Cooker Pork Carnitas (page 186)
Calories: 599; Fat: 44g; Protein: 41g; Total Carbs: 7g; Fiber: 1g; Net Carbs: 6g
68% fat, 27% protein, 5% carbs

DINNER SIDE DISH: Cauliflower Rice (page 218)
Calories: 82; Fat: 4g; Protein: 4g; Total Carbs: 11g; Fiber: 5g; Net Carbs: 6g
44% fat, 20% protein, 36% carbs

MONDAY'S TOTAL NUTRITION
Calories: 1,542; Fat: 114; Protein: 102g; Total Carbs: 28g; Fiber: 9g; Net Carbs: 19g
67% fat, 26% protein, 7% carbs

Tuesday

BREAKFAST: Almond Coconut Hot Cereal (page 58)
Calories: 395; Fat: 36g; Protein: 7g; Total Carbs: 13g; Fiber: 5g; Net Carbs: 8g
82% fat, 7% protein, 11% carbs

LUNCH: Essential Cobb Salad (page 97)
Calories: 500; Fat: 44g; Protein: 16g; Total Carbs: 11g; Fiber: 5g; Net Carbs: 6g
79% fat, 13% protein, 8% carbs

DINNER: Meatloaf (page 180)
Calories: 437; Fat: 34g; Protein: 28g; Total Carbs: 5g; Fiber: 1g; Net Carbs: 4g
70% fat, 26% protein, 4% carbs

DINNER SIDE DISH: Killer Kale Salad (page 91)
Calories: 188; Fat: 14g; Protein: 5g; Total Carbs: 15g; Fiber: 7g; Net Carbs: 8g
67% fat, 11% protein, 22% carbs

TUESDAY'S TOTAL NUTRITION
Calories: 1,520; Fat: 128g; Protein: 56g; Total Carbs: 44g; Fiber: 18g; Net Carbs: 26g
75% fat, 15% protein, 10% carbs

Wednesday

BREAKFAST: Lemon Berry Yogurt Parfait (page 56)
Calories: 331; Fat: 28g; Protein: 13g; Total Carbs: 12g; Fiber: 5g; Net Carbs: 7g
76% fat, 16% protein, 8% carbs

LUNCH: Essential Cobb Salad (page 97)
Calories: 500; Fat: 44g; Protein: 16g; Total Carbs: 11g; Fiber: 5g; Net Carbs: 6g
79% fat, 13% protein, 8% carbs

SNACK/DESSERT: No-Bake Coconut Chocolate Squares (page 203)
Calories: 144; Fat: 16g; Protein: 1g; Total Carbs: 2g; Fiber: 1g; Net Carbs: 1g
98% fat, 1% protein, 1% carbs

DINNER: Chicken Marsala Soup (page 103)
Calories: 429; Fat: 26g; Protein: 38g; Total Carbs: 8g; Fiber: 1g; Net Carbs: 7g
55% fat, 35% protein, 7% carbs

WEDNESDAY'S TOTAL NUTRITION
Calories: 1,404; Fat: 114g; Protein: 68g; Total Carbs: 33g; Fiber: 12g; Net Carbs: 21g
73% fat, 19% protein, 8% carbs

Thursday

BREAKFAST: Broccoli Bacon Egg Muffin Cups (page 66)
Calories: 338; Fat: 22g; Protein: 29g; Total Carbs: 4g; Fiber: 1g; Net Carbs: 3g
62% fat, 34% protein, 4% carbs

LUNCH: Chicken Marsala Soup (page 103)
Calories: 429; Fat: 26g; Protein: 38g; Total Carbs: 8g; Fiber: 1g; Net Carbs: 7g
55% fat, 35% protein, 7% carbs

SNACK: Almond Crackers (page 73)
Calories: 273; Fat: 25g; Protein: 8g; Total Carbs: 8g; Fiber: 4g; Net Carbs: 4g
78% fat, 11% protein, 11% carbs

DINNER: Pepper-Crusted Salmon with Wilted Kale (page 133)
Calories: 442; Fat: 29g; Protein: 37g; Total Carbs: 8g; Fiber: 3g; Net Carbs: 5g
60% fat, 33% protein, 7% carbs

THURSDAY'S TOTAL NUTRITION
Calories: 1,482; Fat: 102g; Protein: 112g; Total Carbs: 28g; Fiber: 9g; Net Carbs: 19g
62% fat, 30% protein, 8% carbs

Friday

BREAKFAST: Almond Coconut Hot Cereal (page 58)
Calories: 395; Fat: 36g; Protein: 7g; Total Carbs: 13g; Fiber: 5g; Net Carbs: 8g
82% fat, 7% protein, 11% carbs

LUNCH: Curried Chicken Salad (page 154)
Calories: 379; Fat: 28g; Protein: 27g; Total Carbs: 4g; Fiber: 1g; Net Carbs: 3g
67% fat, 29% protein, 4% carbs

SNACK/DESSERT: No-Bake Coconut Chocolate Squares (page 203)
Calories: 144; Fat: 16g; Protein: 1g; Total Carbs: 2g; Fiber: 1g; Net Carbs: 1g
98% fat, 1% protein, 1% carbs

DINNER: BBQ Baby Back Ribs (page 189)
Calories: 654; Fat: 51g; Protein: 42g; Total Carbs: 6g; Fiber: 1g; Net Carbs: 5g
70% fat, 26% protein, 4% carbs

FRIDAY'S TOTAL NUTRITION
Calories: 1,572; Fat: 131g; Protein: 77g; Total Carbs: 25g; Fiber: 8g; Net Carbs: 17g
75% fat, 20% protein, 5% carbs

Saturday

BREAKFAST: Chile Relleno Scrambled Eggs (page 65)
Calories: 346; Fat: 31g; Protein: 15g; Total Carbs: 3g; Fiber: 0g; Net Carbs: 3g
81% fat, 16% protein, 3% carbs

LUNCH: BBQ Baby Back Ribs (page 189)
Calories: 654; Fat: 51g; Protein: 42g; Total Carbs: 6g; Fiber: 1g; Net Carbs: 5g
70% fat, 26% protein, 4% carbs

DINNER: Chicken Cordon Bleu (page 164)
Calories: 476; Fat: 31g; Protein: 45g; Total Carbs: 5g; Fiber: 2g; Net Carbs: 3g
59% fat, 37% protein, 4% carbs

DINNER SIDE DISH: Killer Kale Salad (page 91)
Calories: 188; Fat: 14g; Protein: 5g; Total Carbs: 15g; Fiber: 7g; Net Carbs: 8g
67% fat, 11% protein, 22% carbs

SATURDAY'S TOTAL NUTRITION
Calories: 1,664; Fat: 127g; Protein: 107g; Total Carbs: 29g; Fiber: 10g; Net Carbs: 19g
70% fat, 25% protein, 5% carbs

Sunday

BREAKFAST: Broccoli Bacon Egg Muffin Cups (page 66)
Calories: 338; Fat: 22g; Protein: 29g; Total Carbs: 4g; Fiber: 1g; Net Carbs: 3g
62% fat, 34% protein, 4% carbs

LUNCH: Chicken Cordon Bleu (page 164)
Calories: 476; Fat: 31g; Protein: 45g; Total Carbs: 5g; Fiber: 2g; Net Carbs: 3g
59% fat, 37% protein, 4% carbs

LUNCH SIDE DISH: Killer Kale Salad (page 91)
Calories: 188; Fat: 14g; Protein: 5g; Total Carbs: 15g; Fiber: 7g; Net Carbs: 8g
67% fat, 11% protein, 22% carbs

SNACK/DESSERT: No-Bake Coconut Chocolate Squares (page 203)
Calories: 144; Fat: 16g; Protein: 1g; Total Carbs: 2g; Fiber: 1g; Net Carbs: 1g
98% fat, 1% protein, 1% carbs

DINNER: Lemongrass Pork Noodle Bowls (page 192)
Calories: 446; Fat: 25g; Protein: 44g; Total Carbs: 9g; Fiber: 3g; Net Carbs: 6g
50% fat, 39% protein, 11% carbs

SUNDAY'S TOTAL NUTRITION
Calories: 1,592; Fat: 108g; Protein 124g; Total Carbs: 35g; Fiber: 14g; Net Carbs: 21g
61% fat, 31% protein, 8% carbs

Week 2 Shopping List

Canned and Bottled Items

- Beef stock (1½ quarts)
- Chiles, green (4-ounce can)
- Coconut milk (8-ounce can)
- Tomato paste (6-ounce can)

Dairy and Eggs

- Blue cheese crumbles (1 small package)
- Butter (12 ounces)
- Cream cheese (4 ounces)
- Eggs (2 dozen)
- Greek yogurt, whole-milk plain (5-ounce container)
- Parmesan cheese, grated (4 ounces)
- Swiss cheese (4 ounces)

Produce

- Avocado, large (1)
- Basil leaves, fresh (1 bunch)
- Blueberries, fresh (½ cup)
- Carrots (2 medium)
- Cauliflower (1 large head)
- Celery (1 small head)
- Cilantro (1 bunch)
- Garlic (1 head)
- Kale, Lacinato (2 bunches)
- Lemon (1)
- Lemongrass, fresh (1 stalk)
- Lettuce, romaine (2 heads)
- Lime (1)
- Mint leaves, fresh (1 bunch)
- Mushrooms, cremini (2 cups)
- Onions, red (3)
- Onions, yellow (3)
- Orange (1)
- Parsley, fresh (1 bunch)
- Raspberries (¼ cup)
- Rosemary, fresh (1 bunch)
- Serrano pepper (1)
- Tomato, plum (1)
- Tomatoes, grape (½ pint)
- Zucchini, medium (2)

Frozen Foods

- Broccoli florets (1 package)

Meat

- Bacon (16 ounces)
- Beef, ground (1 pound)
- Chicken thighs, boneless, skinless (2 pounds)
- Chicken, white and dark meat (16 ounces)
- Pork shoulder, boneless (1½ pounds)
- Pork tenderloin (1¼ pounds)
- Pork, ground (1 pound)
- Prosciutto or deli ham (4 ounces)
- Salmon (1½ pounds)

Pantry Items

- Almond flour
- Black peppercorns
- Canola oil
- Cashews (¼ cup)
- Cinnamon, ground
- Cinnamon stick (1)
- Cloves, ground
- Cocoa powder, unsweetened
- Coconut oil
- Coconut, unsweetened, shredded (1½ cups)
- Cumin, ground

Pantry Items *(continued)*

- Curry powder
- Dijon mustard
- Extra-virgin olive oil
- Hazelnuts (¼ cup)
- Mayonnaise, full-fat
- Oregano, dried
- Pecans (¼ cup)
- Red wine vinegar
- Sea salt
- Soy sauce, low-sodium
- Stevia, liquid
- Vanilla extract
- White wine vinegar

Other

- Marsala wine

Meal Plan—Week 3

You are amazing! By now, the "keto flu" is likely behind you and you're enjoying continued weight loss and improved energy levels.

The theme for this week is personal responsibility. Begin gathering recipes and crafting your own menus based on the foods you have enjoyed and your personal carb threshold—that is, the number of carbs and fiber that keep you feeling full and energized while still losing weight. Your success is in your hands, and you have all the tools you need to succeed. Use the recipes in this book and beyond to craft menus that you will enjoy.

One pitfall to avoid this week is getting overly confident in your progress and adding carb-rich foods back onto the menu before you have reached your goals. It's not that a few grams of carbs here or there are that devastating to your progress or will instantly stall your ketosis—although too many will. The problem is that they make the diet so much more difficult to stick to. Being in ketosis is about breaking your reliance on quick-burning carbs for energy. Make it easier on yourself by sticking to the plan.

By now, your hunger has likely leveled off and you can go hours between meals without feeling hungry. This is one of the huge payoffs of being in ketosis! Hence, this week does not include many snacks or desserts. If you find yourself hungry between meals, perhaps it is because the daily calorie counts on this menu are lower than your daily caloric needs. In that case, you can have one of the fat bombs from the snacks or desserts category. Alternatively, double up on some of the entrée portions at lunch or dinner.

Monday

BREAKFAST: Peanut Butter Whipped Greek Yogurt (page 57)
Calories: 322; Fat: 22g; Protein: 23g; Total Carbs: 11g; Fiber: 2g; Net Carbs: 9g
61% fat, 28% protein, 11% carbs

LUNCH: Spaghetti Squash Chicken Bowls (page 160)
Calories: 440; Fat: 25g; Protein: 40g; Total Carbs: 13g; Fiber: 2g; Net Carbs: 11g
51% fat, 36% protein, 13% carbs

DINNER: Swedish Meatballs (page 183)
Calories: 509; Fat: 42g; Protein: 29g; Total Carbs: 3g; Fiber: 1g; Net Carbs: 2g
74% fat, 23% protein, 3% carbs

DINNER SIDE DISH: Everyday Caesar Salad (page 89)
Calories: 224; Fat: 22g; Protein: 4g; Total Carbs: 4g; Fiber: 2g; Net Carbs: 2g
88% fat, 7% protein, 5% carbs

MONDAY'S TOTAL NUTRITION

Calories: 1,495; Fat: 111g; Protein: 96g; Total Carbs: 31g; Fiber: 7g; Net Carbs: 23g
67% fat, 26% protein, 7% carbs

Tuesday

BREAKFAST: Bulletproof Pancakes (page 62)
Calories: 365; Fat: 35g; Protein: 10g; Total Carbs: 7g; Fiber: 3g; Net Carbs: 4g
87% fat, 10% protein, 3% carbs

LUNCH: Spaghetti Squash Chicken Bowls (page 160)
Calories: 440; Fat: 25g; Protein: 40g; Total Carbs: 13g; Fiber: 2g; Net Carbs: 11g
51% fat, 36% protein, 13% carbs

DINNER: Halibut in Tomato Basil Sauce (page 135)
Calories: 467; Fat: 31g; Protein: 38g; Total Carbs: 5g; Fiber: 0g; Net Carbs: 5g
60% fat, 33% protein, 7% carbs

DINNER SIDE DISH: Everyday Caesar Salad (page 89)
Calories: 224; Fat: 22g; Protein: 4g; Total Carbs: 4g; Fiber: 2g; Net Carbs: 2g
88% fat, 7% protein, 5% carbs

TUESDAY'S TOTAL NUTRITION

Calories: 1,496; Fat: 113g; Protein: 92g; Total Carbs: 33g; Fiber: 9g; Net Carbs: 24g
68% fat, 24% protein, 8% carbs

Wednesday

BREAKFAST: Roasted Vegetable Hash (page 68)
Calories: 443; Fat: 37g; Protein: 15g; Total Carbs: 16g; Fiber: 4g; Net Carbs: 12g
75% fat, 12% protein, 13% carbs

LUNCH: Halibut in Tomato Basil Sauce (page 135)
Calories: 467; Fat: 31g; Protein: 38g; Total Carbs: 5g; Fiber: 0g; Net Carbs: 5g
60% fat, 33% protein, 7% carbs

SNACK/DESSERT: Key Lime Pie Fat Bombs (page 202)
Calories: 98; Fat: 10g; Protein: 2g; Total Carbs: 3g; Fiber: 1g; Net Carbs: 2g
96% fat, 2% protein, 2% carbs

DINNER: Swedish Meatballs (page 183)
Calories: 509; Fat: 42g; Protein: 29g; Total Carbs: 3g; Fiber: 1g; Net Carbs: 2g
74% fat, 23% protein, 3% carbs

WEDNESDAY'S TOTAL NUTRITION

Calories: 1,517; Fat: 120g; Protein: 84g; Total Carbs: 27g; Fiber: 6g; Net Carbs: 21g
71% fat, 21% protein, 8% carbs

Thursday

BREAKFAST: Bulletproof Pancakes (page 62)
Calories: 365; Fat: 35g; Protein: 10g; Total Carbs: 7g; Fiber: 3g; Net Carbs: 4g
87% fat, 10% protein, 3% carbs

LUNCH: Tuna-Stuffed Avocado (2 Servings) (page 80)
Calories: 550; Fat: 48g; Protein: 20g; Total Carbs: 18g; Fiber: 12g; Net Carbs: 6g
78% fat, 14% protein, 8% carbs

DINNER: Chorizo, Chicken, and Salsa Verde (page 168)
Calories: 661; Fat: 52g; Protein: 40g; Total Carbs: 8g; Fiber: 2g; Net Carbs: 6g
71% fat, 24% protein, 5% carbs

THURSDAY'S TOTAL NUTRITION

Calories: 1,576; Fat: 135g; Protein: 70g; Total Carbs: 33g; Fiber: 17g; Net Carbs: 16g
72% fat, 18% protein, 10% carbs

Friday

BREAKFAST: Peanut Butter Whipped Greek Yogurt (page 57)
Calories: 322; Fat: 22g; Protein: 23g; Total Carbs: 11g; Fiber: 2g; Net Carbs: 9g
61% fat, 28% protein, 11% carbs

LUNCH: Chorizo, Chicken, and Salsa Verde (page 168)
Calories: 661; Fat: 52g; Protein: 40g; Total Carbs: 8g; Fiber: 2g; Net Carbs: 6g
71% fat, 24% protein, 5% carbs

DINNER: Beef Mushroom Stroganoff (page 196)
Calories: 605; Fat: 47g; Protein: 30g; Total Carbs: 7g; Fiber: 1g; Net Carbs: 6g
73% fat, 22% protein, 5% carbs

FRIDAY'S TOTAL NUTRITION

Calories: 1,588; Fat: 121g; Protein: 93g; Total Carbs: 26g; Fiber: 5g; Net Carbs: 21g
70% fat, 23% protein, 7% carbs

Saturday

BREAKFAST: Roasted Vegetable Hash (page 68)
Calories: 443; Fat: 37g; Protein: 15g; Total Carbs: 16g; Fiber: 4g; Net Carbs: 12g
75% fat, 12% protein, 13% carbs

LUNCH: Beef Mushroom Stroganoff (page 196)
Calories: 605; Fat: 47g; Protein: 30g; Total Carbs: 7g; Fiber: 1g; Net Carbs: 6g
73% fat, 22% protein, 5% carbs

DINNER: Roasted Chicken and Zucchini with Wine Reduction (page 151)
Calories: 490; Fat: 34g; Protein: 36g; Total Carbs: 5g; Fiber: 1g; Net Carbs: 4g
64% fat, 32% protein, 4% carbs

SATURDAY'S TOTAL NUTRITION

Calories: 1,538; Fat: 118g; Protein: 81g; Total Carbs: 28g; Fiber: 6g; Net Carbs: 22g
71% fat, 22% protein, 7% carbs

Sunday

BREAKFAST: Dutch Babies (page 63)
Calories: 310; Fat: 22g; Protein: 21g; Total Carbs: 7g; Fiber: 3g; Net Carbs: 4g
64% fat, 27% protein, 9% carbs

LUNCH: Roasted Chicken and Zucchini with Wine Reduction (page 151)
Calories: 490; Fat: 34g; Protein: 36g; Total Carbs: 5g; Fiber: 1g; Net Carbs: 4g
64% fat, 32% protein, 4% carbs

DINNER: Braised Beef Short Ribs (page 187)
Calories: 774; Fat: 65g; Protein: 30g; Total Carbs: 10g; Fiber: 4g; Net Carbs: 6g
76% fat, 16% protein, 8% carbs

SUNDAY'S TOTAL NUTRITION
Calories: 1,574; Fat: 121g; Protein: 87g; Total Carbs: 22g; Fiber: 8g; Net Carbs: 14g
70% fat, 24% protein, 6% carbs

Week 3 Shopping List

Canned and Bottled Items

- Beef stock (1 quart plus 12 ounces)
- Chicken broth, low-sodium (16 ounces)
- Tuna, packed in water (6-ounce can)

Dairy and Eggs

- Butter (12 ounces)
- Eggs (2 dozen)
- Greek yogurt, whole-milk plain (15-ounce container)
- Half-and-half (1 small container)
- Heavy cream (1 small container)
- Milk, whole (1 small container)
- Sour cream (12-ounce container)

Meat

- Beef short ribs (about 1½ pounds)
- Beef, ground (½ pound)
- Chicken thighs, bone-in, skin-on (4½ pounds)
- Chorizo (½ pound)
- Halibut (1¼ pounds)
- Pork, ground (½ pound)
- Steak, rib-eye, well-marbled (1¼ pounds)

Pantry Items

- Allspice, ground
- Almond flour
- Baking soda
- Bay leaves
- Canola oil
- Cashews, roasted
- Chili powder
- Chocolate chips, no sugar added (such as Lily's brand)
- Cinnamon, ground
- Coconut flour
- Coconut oil
- Extra-virgin olive oil
- Mayonnaise, full-fat
- Mustard, whole-grain
- Nutmeg, ground
- Peanut butter, natural
- Red pepper flakes
- Red wine vinegar
- Sesame oil, toasted
- Soy sauce, low-sodium
- Stevia, liquid
- Vanilla extract
- White wine vinegar

Produce

- Avocado (1 large)
- Basil, fresh (1 bunch)
- Bell pepper, green (1)
- Carrots (2)
- Cauliflower (1 large head)
- Celery (4 stalks)
- Cilantro, fresh (1 bunch)
- Garlic (1 head)
- Ginger (1 small piece)
- Jalapeño pepper (1)
- Lemon (1)
- Limes (2)
- Mushrooms, cremini (8 ounces)
- Onion, red (1 small)
- Onions, yellow (4 medium)
- Oregano (1 bunch)
- Parsley, fresh (1 bunch)
- Scallions (1 bunch)
- Shallot (1 small)
- Squash, spaghetti (1 small)
- Thyme, fresh (1 bunch)
- Tomatoes, grape (1 pint)
- Zucchini (3 medium)

Other

- Brandy
- Red wine, dry
- White wine

PART TWO

The Recipes

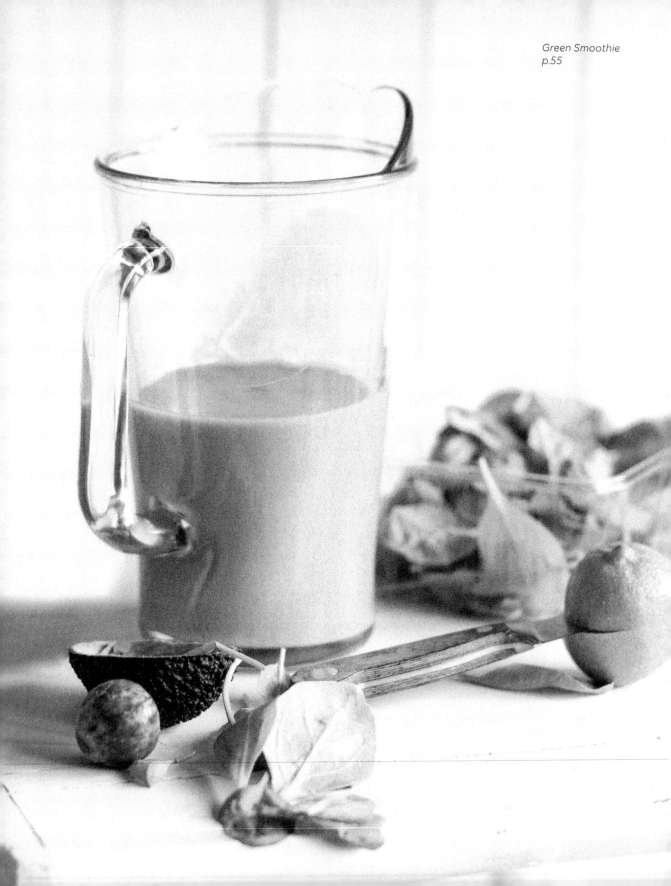

Green Smoothie
p.55

CHAPTER FOUR
Smoothies & Breakfasts

Nutty Chocolate Protein Shake

Serves 1 / Prep time: 5 minutes / Cook time: 0 minutes

DAIRY FREE • VEGETARIAN • 30 MINUTES OR LESS

I could drink this protein shake every day. It's my go-to for busy mornings and is a great alternative to eggs on a low-carb diet. I use unsweetened almond milk because it is low in carbs and calories and is dairy free.

1 cup unsweetened almond milk

1 cup ice

1 tablespoon peanut butter
  or almond butter

1 scoop chocolate protein powder

1. In a blender, blend the almond milk, ice, and peanut butter until smooth.

2. With the blender running, slowly add the protein powder, scraping down the sides with a spatula as needed. Serve immediately.

PER SERVING Calories: 368; Fat: 22g; Protein: 39g; Total Carbs: 12g; Fiber: 6g; Net Carbs: 6g
54% fat, 41% protein, 5% carbs

INGREDIENT TIP: Choose a protein powder sweetened with at least 20 grams of protein and 10 or fewer grams of carbohydrates. My favorite is Vega Sport Protein in chocolate flavor. It is naturally dairy free and sweetened with stevia.

Green Smoothie

Serves 1 / Prep time: 5 minutes / Cook time: 0 minutes

DAIRY FREE • VEGETARIAN • 30 MINUTES OR LESS

This smoothie is packed with healthy greens, vitamins, minerals, and antioxidants. The total carb count might seem high, but it is mostly fiber—10 grams! Don't skimp on the lime juice; it really brightens the flavor.

1 cup unsweetened almond milk

1 cup ice

1 cup spinach

½ cup chopped fresh parsley

½ cup chopped fresh cilantro

½ avocado, pitted and peeled

1 tablespoon lime juice

3 to 4 drops liquid stevia

1. In a blender, add all of the ingredients in order. Pulse the mixture a few times until roughly combined. Scrape down the sides if needed.

2. Blend until smooth, and serve immediately.

PER SERVING Calories: 208; Fat: 16g; Protein: 5g; Total Carbs: 13g; Fiber: 10g; Net Carbs: 3g
70% fat, 10% protein, 20% carbs

INGREDIENT TIP: Use the stems of the herbs in addition to the leaves; most of the flavor is actually in the stems.

Lemon Berry Yogurt Parfait

KETO
QUOTIENT

1 ② 3

Serves 1 / Prep time: 5 minutes / Cook time: 0 minutes

VEGETARIAN • 30 MINUTES OR LESS

Fruit in a low-carb cookbook? Yes, and contrary to popular belief, it doesn't pile on the carbs or the pounds. Fruit gives this simple berry and yogurt parfait some color and flavor while keeping it under 10 grams of net carbs per serving.

5 ounces whole-milk plain
   Greek yogurt
½ teaspoon lemon zest

1 to 2 drops liquid stevia (optional)
¼ cup roughly chopped pecans
¼ cup raspberries

1. In a small bowl, mix together the yogurt, lemon zest, and stevia (if using).

2. Place half of the yogurt into a small glass. Top with half of the raspberries followed by half of the pecans. Repeat with another layer each of yogurt, berries, and pecans. Serve immediately or cover and chill until ready to serve.

PER SERVING Calories: 331; Fat: 28g; Protein: 13g; Total Carbs: 12g; Fiber: 5g; Net Carbs: 7g
76% fat, 16% protein, 8% carbs

VARIATION TIP: Use another low-sugar fruit such as blackberries or strawberries in place of the raspberries if you wish. The pecans can also be replaced with macadamia nuts, walnuts, or pistachios.

Peanut Butter Whipped Greek Yogurt

Serves 1 / Prep time: 5 minutes / Cook time: 0 minutes

VEGETARIAN • 30 MINUTES OR LESS

I can understand if you mistake this decadent breakfast for a dessert. It is smooth and rich with creamy Greek yogurt and peanut butter sweetened with stevia and studded with no-sugar-added chocolate chips. It will quickly become your new go-to low-carb breakfast or snack. Choose natural peanut butter to avoid hydrogenated oils and added sugar.

5 ounces whole-milk plain
Greek yogurt

2 tablespoons creamy natural
peanut butter

1 to 2 drops liquid stevia (optional)

15 no-sugar-added chocolate chips,
such as Lily's brand

1. In a bowl, whisk together the yogurt, peanut butter, and stevia (if using) until light and fluffy.

2. Stir in the chocolate chips.

PER SERVING Calories: 322; Fat: 22g; Protein: 23g; Total Carbs: 11g; Fiber: 2g; Net Carbs: 9g
61% fat, 28% protein, 11% carbs

Almond Coconut Hot Cereal

Serves 1 / Prep time: 5 minutes / Cook time: 1 minute

DAIRY FREE • VEGETARIAN • 30 MINUTES OR LESS

This simple, warming breakfast "cereal" isn't cereal at all. Instead, it's a delicious combination of almond flour and shredded coconut cooked in coconut milk. Make a big batch of the dry ingredients and store in a jar so it's easy to prepare on busy mornings.

¼ cup almond flour

Pinch sea salt

¼ teaspoon ground cinnamon

3 tablespoons unsweetened
   shredded coconut

½ cup coconut milk

1. In a microwave-safe bowl, mix together the almond flour, sea salt, cinnamon, and shredded coconut. Stir in the coconut milk, adding water if necessary to thin to the desired consistency.

2. Microwave on high for 30 seconds. Stir and microwave for another 30 seconds or until heated through.

PER SERVING Calories: 395; Fat: 36g; Protein: 7g; Total Carbs: 13g; Fiber: 5g; Net Carbs: 8g
82% fat, 7% protein, 11% carbs

VARIATION TIP: For added flavor and texture, reserve half of the shredded coconut and toast it in a dry skillet. Top the hot cereal with the toasted coconut just before serving.

Macadamia Nut Granola

Serves 6 / Prep time: 10 minutes / Cook time: 15 minutes

DAIRY FREE • VEGETARIAN • 30 MINUTES OR LESS

This nutty granola will satisfy your cravings for something crunchy without exceeding your daily carb allotment. Make a big batch at the beginning of the week so you'll be able to enjoy it for meals and snacks all week long.

1 cup macadamia nuts

1 cup almonds

1 cup shredded unsweetened coconut

1 egg white, whisked

¼ cup coconut oil, melted

1 teaspoon vanilla extract

½ teaspoon liquid stevia

½ teaspoon sea salt

1. Preheat the oven to 325°F.

2. In a food processor, pulse the macadamia nuts and almonds until the mixture is about the texture of rolled oats. Add the coconut and pulse once or twice to mix.

3. In a separate bowl, mix together the egg white, coconut oil, vanilla, stevia, and sea salt. Pour this over the nut mixture and stir to mix.

4. Spread the granola into an 8-by-8-inch baking dish. Bake for 7 to 8 minutes. Stir and bake for another 7 to 8 minutes until the granola is golden brown. Allow to cool at room temperature before storing in a covered container.

PER SERVING (½ cup) Calories: 466; Fat: 43g; Protein: 8g; Total Carbs: 12g; Fiber: 7g; Net Carbs: 5g; 84% fat, 6% protein, 10% carbs

PER SERVING WITH MILK (½ cup granola and ½ cup whole milk) Calories: 541; Fat: 50g; Protein: 12g; Total Carbs: 18g; Fiber: 7g; Net Carbs: 11g; 82% fat, 8% protein, 10% carbs

VARIATION TIP: Serve ¼ cup of the granola with 5 ounces of Greek yogurt and 2 tablespoons of fresh or frozen blueberries.

VARIATION PER SERVING Calories: 363; Fat: 28g; Protein: 18g; Total Carbs: 13g; Fiber: 4g; Net Carbs: 9g; 69% fat, 20% protein, 11% carbs

Ricotta-Stuffed Crêpes

Serves 4 / Prep time: 5 minutes / Cook time: 10 minutes

VEGETARIAN • 30 MINUTES OR LESS

These luxurious stuffed crêpes remind me of cannoli. But without the deep fryer, wheat, and sugar, this version is actually good for you! See the substitution tip for a dairy-free version.

4 eggs

½ cup almond flour

¼ cup half-and-half

⅛ teaspoon sea salt

1 teaspoon vanilla extract

1 cup whole-milk ricotta cheese

8 to 10 drops liquid stevia

¼ teaspoon ground cinnamon

2 tablespoons butter

1 tablespoon unsweetened
   cocoa powder

1. In a blender, purée the eggs, almond flour, half-and-half, sea salt, and vanilla extract until smooth.

2. In a separate bowl, stir together the ricotta, stevia, and cinnamon. Set aside.

3. Melt ½ tablespoon of the butter in a small nonstick skillet over medium heat. Once the butter is hot, pour in about ¼ of the crêpe batter and swirl to coat the pan. Cook for 1 to 2 minutes, or until the egg is set. Carefully flip the crêpe and cook on the other side for about 30 seconds.

4. Transfer to a separate plate and repeat with the remaining batter, using ½ tablespoon of the butter for each crêpe. You should have four crêpes total.

5. Scoop ¼ cup of the ricotta mixture into the center of each crêpe. Roll each into a cylinder and place on serving plates. Sift the cocoa powder over each crêpe using a fine mesh sieve.

PER SERVING Calories: 293; Fat: 24g; Protein: 15g; Total Carbs: 5g; Fiber: 1g; Net Carbs: 4g 73% fat, 19% protein, 8% carbs

SUBSTITUTION TIP: To make a dairy-free crêpe, use full-fat coconut milk in place of the half-and-half and coat the pan with coconut oil. Skip the ricotta cheese and spoon 1 tablespoon of almond butter on each crêpe.

SUBSTITUTION PER SERVING Calories: 298; Fat: 27g; Protein: 10g; Total Carbs: 6g; Fiber: 3g; Net Carbs: 3g; 80% fat, 13% protein, 7% carbs

Bulletproof Pancakes

Serves 4 / Prep time: 10 minutes / Cook time: 10 minutes

VEGETARIAN • 30 MINUTES OR LESS

You have heard of Bulletproof Coffee (page 217) —now try bulletproof pancakes. Like the beverage, these breakfast staples combine coconut oil and butter for a rich, creamy texture. They're sweetened with stevia; for an extra special treat, drizzle with butter and maybe add some berries.

2 eggs

2 tablespoons coconut oil, melted

¼ cup whole milk

1 teaspoon vanilla extract

8 to 10 drops liquid stevia

¼ teaspoon ground cinnamon

1 cup almond flour

½ teaspoon baking soda

¼ teaspoon sea salt

4 tablespoons butter, divided

1. In a blender, purée the eggs, coconut oil, milk, vanilla extract, stevia, cinnamon, flour, baking soda, and sea salt until smooth. Allow the batter to rest for 5 minutes.

2. Heat about ½ tablespoon of the butter in a large, nonstick skillet over medium heat. Pour ¼ cup of the batter into the pan and cook until the edges are set and bubbles form throughout the pancake, about 2 minutes. Carefully flip and cook on the other side for 1 minute. Repeat with the remaining batter, adding more butter to the pan as needed.

3. Top the cooked pancakes with pats of the remaining butter and serve.

PER SERVING (two 4-inch pancakes) Calories: 365; Fat: 35g; Protein: 10g; Total Carbs: 7g; Fiber: 3g; Net Carbs: 4g; 87% fat, 10% protein, 3% carbs

PREP TIP: Freeze leftover pancakes and store in a zip-top bag until ready to use. Reheat in the toaster oven or microwave.

Dutch Babies

Serves 4 / Prep time: 5 minutes / Cook time: 18 to 20 minutes

NUT FREE • VEGETARIAN • 30 MINUTES OR LESS

These oven pancakes are a staple in my kitchen, and the kids are over-joyed when they appear on the breakfast table. They puff up gloriously in the oven, making them feel like an extra special treat. Serve with butter or top with thinly sliced apples before baking.

12 eggs

½ cup half-and-half

1 tablespoon vanilla extract

8 to 10 drops liquid stevia

¼ cup coconut flour

⅛ teaspoon sea salt

1 tablespoon butter

1. Preheat the oven to 400°F.

2. In a blender, purée the eggs, half-and-half, vanilla extract, stevia, coconut flour, and sea salt until smooth.

3. In a large, ovenproof skillet, such as a cast iron skillet, melt the butter over medium-high heat until hot and bubbling.

4. Pour the batter into the pan and carefully transfer it to the oven. Bake for 18 to 20 minutes, or until the top is golden brown and puffy.

PER SERVING Calories: 310; Fat: 22g; Protein: 21g; Total Carbs: 7g; Fiber: 3g; Net Carbs: 4g 64% fat, 27% protein, 9% carbs

VARIATION TIP: Thinly slice one ripe pear with skin and arrange it on the top of the batter in a circular pattern. Sprinkle with ¼ teaspoon of ground cinnamon or nutmeg. Bake as directed.

VARIATION PER SERVING Calories: 331; Fat: 22g; Protein: 21g; Total Carbs: 13g; Fiber: 4g; Net Carbs: 9g; 64% fat, 27% protein, 9% carbs

Ham and Cheese Egg Scramble

KETO
QUOTIENT

1 ② 3

Serves 1 / Prep time: 5 minutes / Cook time: 5 minutes

NUT FREE • 30 MINUTES OR LESS

Eggs, ham, and cheese are a classic flavor combination in this savory breakfast scramble. You can also use sausage or bacon in the recipe, but I prefer the convenience of cooked ham.

1 tablespoon butter

2 eggs, whisked

Sea salt

Freshly ground black pepper

2 tablespoons diced ham

2 tablespoons shredded pepper
    Jack cheese

½ avocado, pitted, peeled,
    and thinly sliced

¼ cup diced tomatoes

1. Melt the butter in a small skillet over medium heat.

2. Add the eggs to the pan and season with salt and pepper. Stir in a circular pattern with a spatula for 3 to 4 minutes, or until nearly set.

3. Stir in the ham and cheese, and stir just until the eggs are set and the cheese begins to melt, about 1 minute.

4. Top with sliced avocado and tomatoes.

PER SERVING Calories: 546; Fat: 47g; Protein: 25g; Total Carbs: 11g; Fiber: 6g; Net Carbs: 5g
77% fat, 18% protein, 5% carbs

Chile Relleno Scrambled Eggs

Serves 1 / Prep time: 5 minutes / Cook time: 5 minutes

NUT FREE • VEGETARIAN • 30 MINUTES OR LESS

Chile Relleno is one of my favorite dishes at Mexican restaurants. This recipe takes all of those delicious flavors and incorporates them into scrambled eggs. Unlike the dish for which it's named, this recipe doesn't require batter and deep-frying, so it's much healthier, too. Use a smaller amount of the green chiles if you like your food less spicy.

1 tablespoon butter

2 eggs, whisked

Pinch sea salt

1 tablespoon chopped green chiles

1 ounce cream cheese,
    cut into ½-inch pieces

1 tablespoon minced fresh cilantro

1. Melt the butter in a small skillet over medium heat.

2. Add the eggs, salt, and chiles to the pan and stir in a circular pattern with a spatula for 3 to 4 minutes, or until nearly set.

3. Stir in the cream cheese, and stir just until the eggs are set and the cream cheese begins to melt, about 1 minute.

4. Top with cilantro.

PER SERVING Calories: 346; Fat: 31g; Protein: 15g; Total Carbs: 3g; Fiber: 0g; Net Carbs: 3g
81% fat, 16% protein, 3% carbs

SUBSTITUTION TIP: For a more authentic flavor, use queso fresco, a semisoft Mexican cheese, in place of the cream cheese. You can usually find queso fresco in the cheese section of well-stocked grocery stores.

Broccoli Bacon Egg Muffin Cups

Serves 4 / Prep time: 10 minutes / Cook time: 15 minutes

DAIRY FREE • NUT FREE • 30 MINUTES OR LESS

This is one of my family's favorite road trip breakfasts. I prepare the ingredients the night before and simply bake in the morning before we leave for our trip.

12 eggs

Sea salt

Freshly ground black pepper

1 cup cooked broccoli florets

8 ounces bacon, cooked
   and crumbled

1. Preheat the oven to 350°F. Line a muffin tin with parchment paper liners.

2. In a large glass measuring cup or pitcher, whisk the eggs. Season with salt and pepper.

3. Divide the broccoli and cooked bacon among the muffin cups.

4. Pour the egg mixture into each of the muffin cups. Carefully transfer the pan to the oven and bake for 15 minutes, or until the eggs are set.

PER SERVING Calories: 338; Fat: 22g; Protein: 29g; Total Carbs: 4g; Fiber: 1g; Net Carbs: 3g
62% fat, 34% protein, 4% carbs

PREP TIP: Parchment paper liners are preferable to traditional paper liners because the egg releases easily from the parchment.

VARIATION TIP: To make a vegetarian version, swap the broccoli and bacon for ¼ cup sun-dried tomatoes, 1 cup shredded spinach, and 4 ounces of crumbled feta cheese.

VARIATION PER SERVING Calories: 301; Fat: 21g; Protein: 24g; Total Carbs: 5g; Fiber: 1g; Net Carbs: 4g; 63% fat, 31% protein, 6% carbs

Loaded Denver Omelet

NUT FREE • 30 MINUTES OR LESS

KETO
QUOTIENT

1 ② 3

If you're not creative, low-carb diets can easily become monochromatic. This gorgeous omelet introduces a splash of color and a hefty dose of flavor to your diet. For a vegetarian version, swap the ham for sliced avocado.

1 tablespoon butter

3 eggs

Sea salt

Freshly ground black pepper

2 tablespoons diced ham

1 scallion, thinly sliced

¼ bell pepper, seeds and ribs removed, thinly sliced

2 tablespoons shredded cheddar cheese

1. Melt the butter in a small nonstick skillet over medium heat.

2. Whisk the eggs in a glass measuring cup and season with salt and pepper.

3. Pour the eggs into the pan and cook for 1 to 2 minutes, or until barely set around the edges. Lift up the edges with a spatula and tilt the pan so that the liquid eggs can slide to the underside of the omelet. Do this on all sides of the omelet.

4. Sprinkle the ham, scallion, bell pepper, and shredded cheese over the eggs and continue cooking for another minute. Fold the omelet in half and cook for 1 minute. Flip carefully and cook for 1 more minute or until the center of the omelet is no longer watery.

PER SERVING Calories: 415; Fat: 33g; Protein: 26g; Total Carbs: 4g; Fiber: 0g; Net Carbs: 4g
72% fat, 25% protein, 3% carbs

PREP TIP: Save time by slicing and dicing the ingredients the night before.

Roasted Vegetable Hash

Serves 1 / Prep time: 10 minutes / Cook time: 15 minutes

DAIRY FREE • NUT FREE • VEGETARIAN • 30 MINUTES OR LESS

Colorful vegetables make a filling low-carb breakfast. It can be made in a skillet on the stove top, or if you feel like feeding a crowd, multiply the ingredients by each additional person and spread them out on a baking sheet to roast in the oven. If you're serving a family who wants a few more carbs, add diced potatoes and sweet potatoes to their servings.

2 tablespoons coconut oil, divided

1 cup diced zucchini

½ cup diced green bell pepper

¼ cup diced red onion

Sea salt

Freshly ground black pepper

1 tablespoon minced fresh parsley

2 eggs

1. Heat 1 tablespoon of the coconut oil in a large skillet over medium-high heat. Season the zucchini, bell pepper, and onion with salt and pepper, and sauté until the vegetables are crisp tender, about 5 minutes. Transfer them to a serving plate and sprinkle with the parsley.

2. In the same skillet, heat the remaining tablespoon of coconut oil. When hot, crack the eggs into the pan, season with salt and pepper, and cook for 3 to 4 minutes, or until the whites are set and the yolks are still runny or reach the desired level of doneness. Set them on top of the vegetable hash.

PER SERVING Calories: 443 Fat: 37g; Protein: 15g; Total Carbs: 16g; Fiber: 4g; Net Carbs: 12g
75% fat, 12% protein, 13% carbs

Breakfast Pizza

Serves 4 / Prep time: 10 minutes / Cook time: 20 minutes

30 MINUTES OR LESS

This dish is part frittata, part pizza. You can top it with whichever vegetables, cheese, and herbs suit your taste and imagination.

4 ounces Italian sausage

8 eggs

½ cup half-and-half

½ cup almond flour

¼ teaspoon sea salt

Freshly ground black pepper

1 cup sliced roasted red bell peppers

1 cup shredded mozzarella cheese

1 tablespoon minced fresh oregano
   (optional)

1. Preheat the oven to 400°F.

2. In a large cast iron or other ovenproof skillet, cook the sausage over medium heat until barely cooked through. Transfer to a separate dish.

3. In a blender, combine the eggs, half-and-half, almond flour, salt, and pepper. Blend until smooth.

4. Pour the egg mixture into the skillet and cook over medium heat for 5 minutes. The sides of the egg mixture will begin to set.

5. Top with the cooked sausage, red bell peppers, mozzarella cheese, and oregano (if using). Transfer the skillet to the oven and bake for 12 to 15 minutes, or until the eggs are completely set.

PER SERVING Calories: 431; Fat: 32g; Protein: 27g; Total Carbs: 8g; Fiber: 2g; Net Carbs: 6g
67% fat, 25% protein, 8% carbs

PREP TIP: Prepare this breakfast pizza in advance and chill it covered in the refrigerator. Then cut it into quarters and freeze individual slices to reheat in the mornings to save time.

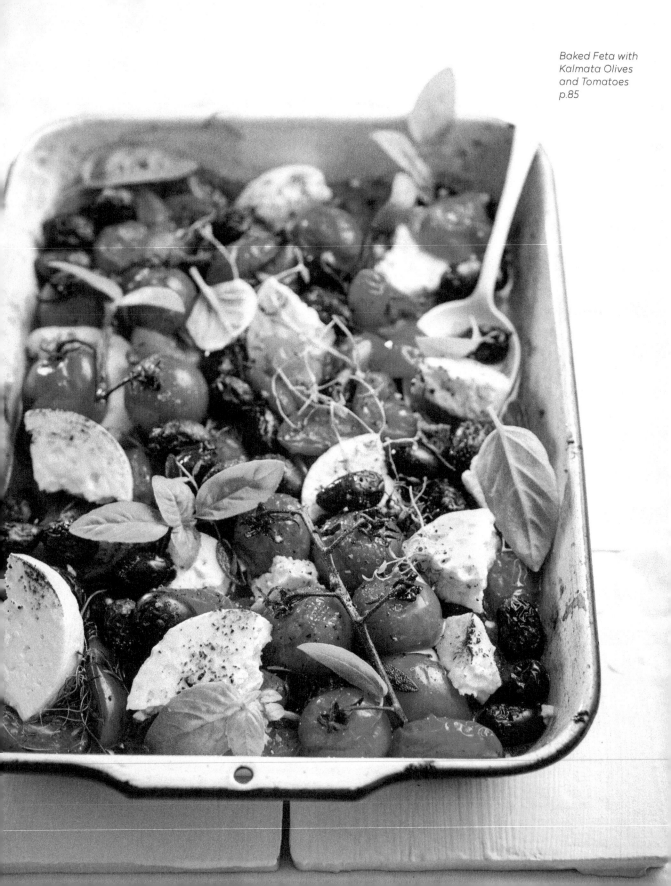

Baked Feta with Kalmata Olives and Tomatoes p.85

CHAPTER FIVE
Snacks & Starters

Parmesan Crisps

KETO
QUOTIENT
① 2 3

Serves 4 / Prep time: 5 minutes / Cook time: 5 minutes

NUT FREE • VEGETARIAN • 30 MINUTES OR LESS

Baked Parmesan makes for a crunchy chip that will satisfy your cravings for something salty and crispy. With just one ingredient, minor prep, and five minutes of baking, this recipe is so easy that it almost feels like cheating.

1 cup grated Parmesan cheese

1. Preheat the oven to 400°F.

2. Line a rimmed baking sheet with parchment paper or use a silicone baking mat.

3. Scoop 1 tablespoon of the Parmesan cheese onto the baking sheet or baking mat with a measuring spoon and flatten gently with the back of the spoon. Repeat with the remaining cheese to create a total of 16 mounds, allowing a couple inches between each mound.

4. Bake for 4 to 5 minutes, or until the cheese is completely melted and beginning to bubble. Allow to cool completely before enjoying or storing in a covered container.

PER SERVING (4 crisps) Calories: 114; Fat: 8g; Protein: 10g; Total Carbs: 1g; Fiber: 0g; Net Carbs: 0g; 70% fat, 30% protein, 0% carbs

INGREDIENT TIP: Use a good quality freshly grated Parmesan cheese rather than the type you shake out of a container for the best results.

Almond Crackers

Serves 6 / Prep time: 5 minutes / Cook time: 10 to 12 minutes

DAIRY FREE • VEGETARIAN • 30 MINUTES OR LESS

These crackers serve as a nice stand-alone snack or a perfect vehicle for creamy dips, cured meat, or cheese. Be careful not to overbake them—they quickly go from golden brown to burnt to a crisp!

2 cups almond flour

½ teaspoon sea salt

3 tablespoons olive oil

1 to 2 tablespoons ice water

1. Preheat the oven to 325°F.

2. In a bowl, stir together the almond flour and sea salt. Stir in the olive oil and just enough water to bind, starting with 1 tablespoon and adding more as needed. Stir until the dough comes together into a ball.

3. Place the ball between two sheets of parchment paper and roll with a rolling pin until very thin, about the thickness of a nickel. Remove the top sheet of parchment paper. Slice the dough into individual squares or rectangles. Carefully slide the dough and parchment paper onto a rimmed baking sheet.

4. Bake for 10 to 12 minutes, or until the crackers are golden brown and crisp. Allow to cool before storing in a covered container.

PER SERVING (2 crackers) Calories: 273; Fat: 25g; Protein: 8g; Total Carbs: 8g; Fiber: 4g; Net Carbs: 4g; 78% fat, 11% protein, 11% carbs

VARIATION TIP: Add 1 tablespoon of fresh herbs such as rosemary, tarragon, or thyme to the dough. They're also delicious with ¼ cup grated Parmesan cheese (but keep in mind that this will change the nutrition information and macros).

Turkey Spinach Rollups

Serves 1 / Prep time: 5 minutes / Cook time: 0 minutes

NUT FREE • 30 MINUTES OR LESS

This simple snack can be added to a big green salad to make a complete meal. Or prepare it up to a day in advance and stash in the refrigerator for when cravings strike.

4 slices (2 ounces) deli
   turkey breast

4 tablespoons cream cheese

¼ cup thinly sliced fresh spinach

2 tablespoons thinly sliced fresh basil
   (optional)

1. Lay one slice of the turkey on a cutting board. Top with 1 tablespoon of the cream cheese, a quarter of the spinach, and ½ tablespoon of the basil (if using).

2. Roll the meat around the filling into a tight cylinder.

3. Repeat with the remaining turkey, cream cheese, spinach, and basil.

PER SERVING Calories: 260; Fat: 21g; Protein: 14g; Total Carbs: 5g; Fiber: 0g; Net Carbs: 5g
73% fat, 22% protein, 5% carbs

VARIATION TIP: Any lunchmeat will work in this easy snack. Swap the turkey for ham, roast beef, or even cheese if you prefer.

Caprese Skewers

NUT FREE • VEGETARIAN • 30 MINUTES OR LESS

KETO QUOTIENT

1 2 3

Caprese salad includes slices of fresh mozzarella layered with ripe tomatoes and showered in fresh basil, olive oil, and balsamic vinegar. It's gorgeous to look at, but sometimes you don't have the time to sit down to a gourmet meal. These skewers offer an on-the-go alternative. They're fewer than 100 calories and so much healthier than the carb-loaded snack packs.

12 small mozzarella balls, about 1 ounce

12 grape tomatoes

12 small basil leaves

Alternating between the ingredients, thread six mozzarella balls, six tomatoes, and six basil leaves onto a bamboo skewer. Repeat with the remaining ingredients on a second skewer. Refrigerate until ready to serve.

PER SERVING Calories: 97; Fat: 5g; Protein: 5g; Total Carbs: 6g; Fiber: 0g; Net Carbs: 6g
46% fat, 21% protein, 21% carbs

VARIATION TIP: To make this into a full meal, double the recipe and place all of the ingredients in a salad bowl. Drizzle with olive oil and balsamic vinegar (but keep in mind that this will change the nutrition information and macros).

Peanut Butter Cookie Dough
Fat Bombs

Serves 8 / Prep time: 5 minutes / Cook time: 0 minutes

VEGETARIAN • 30 MINUTES OR LESS

If you like eating cookie dough but aren't too keen on blowing all your carbs for the week (or risking salmonella from uncooked eggs), try these delicious peanut butter cookie dough bites. They're a good source of fat to keep you in ketosis and they taste like a treat, so dieting doesn't feel like deprivation.

½ cup natural peanut butter

4 tablespoons coconut oil, melted

4 tablespoons butter, at room
   temperature

6 to 7 drops liquid stevia

Pinch sea salt

1. In a small mixing bowl, mix together all of the ingredients.

2. Scoop 1 tablespoon of the mixture into a mini muffin paper, repeating until all the dough is used.

3. Place the bombs in a covered container in the refrigerator and allow them to firm up for at least 30 minutes. These will keep for up to one week in the refrigerator.

PER SERVING Calories: 215; Fat: 21g; Protein: 4g; Total Carbs: 3g; Fiber: 1g; Net Carbs: 2g
88% fat, 7% protein, 5% carbs

VARIATION TIP: To make these seem more like peanut butter cookies, roll the individual balls in crushed dry-roasted peanuts, sea salt, and a granulated-sugar alternative, and flatten with the palm of your hand.

Bacon Chive Fat Bombs

Serves 8 / Prep time: 5 minutes / Cook time: 0 minutes

NUT FREE • 30 MINUTES OR LESS

When you need more calories and fat but don't want any extra carbs, fat bombs are your secret weapon. As the name of this recipe suggests, these savory morsels are loaded with fat. They're also loaded with flavor thanks to cooked bacon and minced fresh chives. Think of them like sour cream and chive potato chips—minus the potatoes!

8 ounces full-fat cream cheese, at room temperature

¼ cup butter, at room temperature

4 slices bacon, cooked, cooled, and crumbled

1 tablespoon minced chives

¼ teaspoon freshly ground black pepper

¼ cup grated Parmesan cheese

1. In a bowl, mix together the cream cheese, butter, crumbled bacon, chives, and pepper.

2. Divide the mixture into eight small balls.

3. Roll the balls in the Parmesan cheese to coat lightly. Refrigerate until ready to serve.

PER SERVING Calories: 190; Fat: 19g; Protein: 5g; Total Carbs: 1g; Fiber: 0g; Net Carbs: 1g
90% fat, 9% protein, 1% carbs

INGREDIENT TIP: Freshly grated Parmesan cheese is usually preferable, but in this case, the shaker variety works well because it is especially dry and forms a light crust on the fat bombs.

Sun-Dried Tomato and Feta Fat Bombs

Serves 8 / Prep time: 5 minutes / Cook time: 0 minutes

VEGETARIAN • 30 MINUTES OR LESS

Tangy sun-dried tomatoes and feta cheese make these fat bombs a delicious alternative to the Bacon Chive Fat Bombs (page 77). Use dry sun-dried tomatoes in this recipe; they are easier to mix into the cheese than sun-dried tomatoes in oil.

4 ounces full-fat cream cheese, at room temperature

¼ cup butter, at room temperature

2 ounces crumbled feta cheese

¼ cup minced sun-dried tomatoes

1 tablespoon minced fresh oregano

1 tablespoon minced fresh parsley

¼ teaspoon freshly ground black pepper

¼ cup almond flour

1. In a bowl, mix together the cream cheese, butter, feta cheese, sun-dried tomatoes, oregano, parsley, and pepper.

2. Divide the mixture into 8 small balls.

3. Roll the balls in the almond flour to coat lightly. Refrigerate until ready to serve.

PER SERVING Calories: 154; Fat: 15g; Protein: 4g; Total Carbs: 3g; Fiber: 1g; Net Carbs: 2g
88% fat, 10% protein, 2% carbs

PREP TIP: To keep the almond flour from getting soggy, wait until just before serving to roll the balls in it.

Fennel and Orange Marinated Olives

Serves 12 / Prep time: 10 minutes / Cook time: 2 hours

DAIRY FREE • VEGETARIAN

If you think low-carb diets are all about deprivation, you are in for a surprise. This marinated olive dish is bursting with the flavors of orange, rosemary, and fennel. Make a large batch for sharing or store it in the refrigerator to enjoy throughout the week. Try to get Marcona almonds, which are crisper than other types.

1 pound Spanish olives with pits

1 cup almonds, preferably Marcona

¾ cup extra-virgin olive oil

1 orange, peeled and very thinly sliced

½ fennel bulb, thinly sliced

1 small red onion, thinly sliced

1 sprig fresh rosemary

1 pinch red pepper flakes

2 tablespoons red wine vinegar

1. Preheat the oven to 300°F.

2. In a shallow baking dish, toss together all of the ingredients. Cover with foil and bake for 1½ hours. Remove the foil and continue baking for another 20 to 30 minutes.

3. Allow the mixture to cool to room temperature before serving.

PER SERVING (about ⅓ cup) Calories: 243; Fat: 24g; Protein: 3g; Total Carbs: 7g; Fiber: 3g; Net Carbs: 4g; 85% fat, 5% protein, 10% carbs

INGREDIENT TIP: When all the olives are gone, the leftover oil makes an awesome salad dressing.

Tuna-Stuffed Avocado

Serves 2 / Prep time: 5 minutes / Cook time: 0 minutes

DAIRY FREE • NUT FREE • 30 MINUTES OR LESS

This tasty snack yields two servings, and leftovers can easily be stored in the refrigerator. Simply keep the avocado and tuna salad separate until ready to serve. Or enjoy the whole thing for a hearty lunch.

3 ounces canned tuna packed
  in water and drained
2 tablespoons full-fat mayonnaise
¼ cup minced celery

1 tablespoon minced shallot
Sea salt
Freshly ground black pepper
1 large avocado, halved and pitted

1. In a small bowl, mix together the tuna, mayonnaise, celery, and shallot. Season with salt and pepper.

2. Spoon about half of the tuna mixture into each avocado half. Serve immediately.

PER SERVING Calories: 275; Fat: 24g; Protein: 10g; Total Carbs: 9g; Fiber: 6g; Net Carbs: 3g
78% fat, 14% protein, 8% carbs

Smoked Salmon and Cucumber Bites

Serves 2 / Prep time: 10 minutes / Cook time: 0 minutes

NUT FREE • 30 MINUTES OR LESS

My best friend, Marcella, made a version of these bites for my bridal shower. She served the smoked salmon atop kettle chips, but it's equally good over sliced cucumber.

½ English cucumber, cut into
  8 to 12 slices

4 ounces cold smoked salmon or lox

½ cup full-fat sour cream

5 sprigs fresh dill, roughly chopped

Freshly ground black pepper

Top each cucumber slice with a small piece of the salmon and a generous spoonful of sour cream. Garnish with a pinch of fresh dill over the sour cream. Season with pepper.

PER SERVING Calories: 179; Fat: 13g; Protein: 12g; Total Carbs: 4g; Fiber: 1g; Net Carbs: 3g
65% fat, 27% protein, 8% carbs

INGREDIENT TIP: Cold smoked salmon or lox is the best choice for this recipe because it does not flake into pieces like home-cooked salmon would.

Tzatziki Dip with Vegetables

Serves 4 / Prep time: 5 minutes / Cook time: 0 minutes

NUT FREE • VEGETARIAN • 30 MINUTES OR LESS

I love vegetables more than most people, but sometimes they need a little sauce or artful preparation to make them sing. This cooling dip does the trick.

5 ounces whole-milk plain
   Greek yogurt

¼ cup full-fat mayonnaise

½ cup diced, peeled cucumbers

1 teaspoon minced fresh dill

1 teaspoon minced fresh garlic

Sea salt

Freshly ground black pepper

4 celery stalks, halved and sliced
   into 3-inch pieces

2 carrots, halved and sliced
   into 3-inch pieces

In a small bowl, mix together the yogurt, mayonnaise, cucumbers, dill, and garlic. Season to taste with salt and pepper. Serve alongside the vegetables.

PER SERVING (¼ cup dip and 6 to 8 vegetable pieces) Calories: 162; Fat: 14g; Protein: 3g; Total Carbs: 9g; Fiber: 2g; Net Carbs: 7g; 78% fat, 7% protein, 15% carbs

VARIATION TIP: Use whatever non-starchy raw vegetables you prefer or have on hand, such as blanched green beans, asparagus, radishes, or grape tomatoes.

Thai Chicken Skewers
with Peanut Sauce

KETO
QUOTIENT

① 2 3

Serves 4 / Prep time: 10 minutes / Cook time: 12 to 15 minutes

DAIRY FREE • 30 MINUTES OR LESS

These skewers are delicious baked, but if you have access to an outdoor grill, fire it up. To make this a complete meal, serve the skewers over a bed of shredded cabbage and top with scallions and cilantro.

1 pound boneless, skinless
   chicken thighs
1 tablespoon toasted sesame oil
Sea salt
Freshly ground black pepper
⅓ cup natural peanut butter

2 tablespoons low-sodium
   soy sauce
Juice of 1 lime
1 teaspoon minced ginger
1 teaspoon minced garlic
Pinch red pepper flakes

1. Preheat the oven to 400°F.

2. Slice the chicken lengthwise into 2-inch-long pieces. Thread the chicken pieces onto four bamboo skewers. Brush the skewered chicken with the sesame oil and season with salt and pepper.

3. Bake for 12 to 15 minutes, or until the chicken is cooked through to an internal temperature of 165°F.

4. Meanwhile, combine the peanut butter, soy sauce, lime juice, ginger, garlic, and red pepper flakes in a small jar. Cover tightly with a lid and shake vigorously. Thin with 2 to 3 tablespoons of water until the sauce reaches the desired consistency.

5. Serve each skewer with 2 tablespoons of the peanut sauce on the side.

PER SERVING (1 skewer) Calories: 316; Fat: 20g; Protein: 31g; Total Carbs: 5g; Fiber: 1g; Net Carbs: 4g; 57% fat, 39% protein, 4% carbs

PREP TIP: There is no need to soak the skewers in water beforehand to keep them from catching fire in the oven or on the grill. Doing so will only make the food soggy.

Prosciutto-Wrapped Mozzarella

Serves 4 / Prep time: 10 minutes / Cook time: 0 minutes

NUT FREE • 30 MINUTES OR LESS

Ham and cheese never looked so gourmet! Prosciutto is a cured meat with a complex, subtle flavor that is almost incomparable to processed deli ham. It works especially well in this simple appetizer because unlike bacon, it does not need to be cooked.

8 slices (4 ounces) prosciutto

16 small bocconcini

1 teaspoon minced rosemary

Freshly ground black pepper

1. Slice the prosciutto in half lengthwise. Wrap one slice of prosciutto around each of the bocconcini and secure with a toothpick.

2. Set the balls on a serving platter and sprinkle with the rosemary and pepper.

PER SERVING (4 balls) Calories: 170; Fat: 14g; Protein: 13g; Total Carbs: 1g; Fiber: 0g; Net Carbs: 1g; 72% fat, 26% protein, 2% carbs

INGREDIENT TIP: Bocconcini are small balls of fresh mozzarella stored in brine. You can find them in most grocery stores alongside other gourmet cheeses or in the deli section.

Baked Feta with Kalamata Olives and Tomatoes

Serves 8 / Prep time: 5 minutes / Cook time: 20 minutes

NUT FREE • VEGETARIAN • 30 MINUTES OR LESS

Feta cheese has a briny taste and becomes soft and creamy when baked. It's especially good over low-carb Almond Crackers (page 73) and perfect as a party appetizer—no one will suspect it's low carb! For an especially beautiful presentation, use vine-ripened cherry tomatoes that still have small pieces of the stem on them.

2 (8-ounce) blocks of feta cheese

1 pint grape or cherry tomatoes

6 ounces Kalamata olives

2 tablespoons roughly chopped fresh oregano

1 lemon, cut into wedges

2 tablespoons extra-virgin olive oil

Sea salt

Freshly ground black pepper

Handful fresh basil leaves, for garnish

1. Preheat the oven to 300°F.

2. Place the feta blocks side by side in a rectangular baking dish. Top with the tomatoes, olives, oregano, and lemon wedges. Drizzle with the olive oil and season with salt and pepper.

3. Bake for 20 minutes, or until the cheese is warmed through and the tomatoes are soft. Squeeze the baked lemon wedges over the dish and top with the fresh basil leaves before serving.

PER SERVING Calories: 207; Fat: 18g; Protein: 8g; Total Carbs: 5g; Fiber: 0g; Net Carbs: 5g
78% fat, 15% protein, 7% carbs

PREP TIP: To make single-serving versions of this dish, divide the feta cheese among eight ramekins (small single-size baking dishes) and top each with a portion of the tomatoes, olives, herbs, and oil. Store the ramekins, tightly covered, in the refrigerator until ready to cook and serve. Bake the filled ramekin in a preheated 300°F oven for 12 minutes.

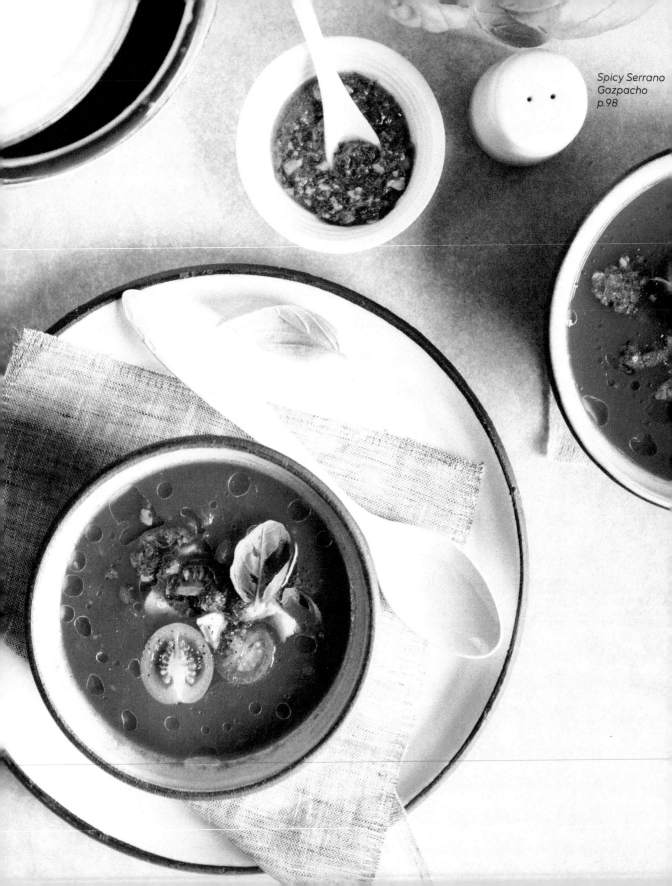

Spicy Serrano
Gazpacho
p.98

CHAPTER SIX
Soups & Salads

Cucumber, Tomato, and Avocado Salad

Serves 4 / Prep time: 10 minutes / Cook time: 0 minutes

DAIRY FREE • NUT FREE • VEGETARIAN • 30 MINUTES OR LESS

I like to make this flavorful salad in the late summer when tomatoes and California avocados are in season.

1 cup halved cherry tomatoes

1 cup diced cucumber

2 large avocados, pitted, peeled, and cut into ½-inch pieces

1 shallot, thinly sliced

2 tablespoons extra-virgin olive oil

2 tablespoons red wine vinegar

Sea salt

Freshly ground black pepper

1. In a medium serving bowl, toss together the tomatoes, cucumber, avocados, and shallot.

2. In a separate container, whisk together the olive oil, vinegar, salt, and pepper. Pour the dressing over the salad.

PER SERVING Calories: 221; Fat: 20g; Protein: 2g; Total Carbs: 11g; Fiber: 7g; Net Carbs: 4g
78% fat, 2% protein, 20% carbs

PREP TIP: Prepare the salad up to 1 hour ahead of time and allow it to rest at room temperature to allow the flavors to come together.

Everyday Caesar Salad

Serves 4 / Prep time: 10 minutes / Cook time: 0 minutes

NUT FREE • 30 MINUTES OR LESS

The restaurant classic you've come to love can now be made at home, and now that fat is back on the menu, you can savor every bite of this creamy, tangy dressing. To make it a complete meal, top it with 4 to 6 ounces of pan-seared salmon or chicken.

⅓ cup full-fat mayonnaise

2 tablespoons extra-virgin olive oil

1 tablespoon lemon juice

1 garlic clove, minced

1 teaspoon anchovy paste (optional)

1 teaspoon Worcestershire sauce

1 teaspoon Dijon mustard

8 cups chopped romaine lettuce

¼ cup grated Parmesan cheese

1. In a large bowl, whisk together the mayonnaise, olive oil, lemon juice, garlic, anchovy paste (if using), Worcestershire sauce, and mustard.

2. Add the romaine lettuce to the bowl, and using clean hands, toss to coat the lettuce in the dressing.

3. Divide the salad among four serving plates and sprinkle a tablespoon of Parmesan cheese over each salad.

PER SERVING Calories: 224; Fat: 22g; Protein: 4g; Total Carbs: 4g; Fiber: 2g; Net Carbs: 2g
88% fat, 7% protein, 5% carbs

PREP TIP: Make the dressing ahead of time and store in a covered container in the refrigerator for up to three days. One serving is approximately 2 tablespoons.

Creamy Broccoli Salad

Serves 4 / Prep time: 10 minutes / Cook time: 10 minutes

DAIRY FREE • NUT FREE • 30 MINUTES OR LESS

Broccoli salads often contain bacon, but they don't always have that delicious bacon fat whisked into the dressing. This version makes the most of the pan drippings to create a luscious, flavorful dressing.

2 slices of applewood smoked bacon,
   cut into pieces
½ cup full-fat mayonnaise
Juice of 1 lemon
Sea salt

Freshly ground black pepper
4 cups raw broccoli florets
½ small red onion, thinly sliced
1 cup shredded red cabbage

1. Cook the bacon in a medium skillet over medium-low heat until the bacon is crisp and has rendered most of its fat. Set the cooked bacon aside.

2. In a large salad bowl, whisk together the bacon fat, mayonnaise, and lemon juice. Season with salt and pepper.

3. Add the broccoli, onion, and red cabbage to the bowl, and mix well. Sprinkle the bacon pieces over the salad just before serving.

PER SERVING Calories: 251; Fat: 23g; Protein: 5g; Total Carbs: 9g; Fiber: 4g; Net Carbs: 5g
82% fat, 8% protein, 10% carbs

VARIATION TIP: The traditional version of this salad is packed with carbs in the form of sugary dried cranberries or raisins. If you're craving a little something sweet, add ¼ cup of diced apple to the salad just before serving for an extra 1 gram of carbohydrates per serving.

Killer Kale Salad

Serves 4 / Prep time: 5 minutes / Cook time: 0 minutes

DAIRY FREE • NUT FREE • VEGETARIAN • 30 MINUTES OR LESS

KETO
QUOTIENT

 2 3

Half of the carbs in this dark, leafy green salad are in the form of fiber, making them indigestible for energy but helpful for keeping your digestive system healthy. Moreover, kale is loaded with beneficial anti-oxidants, vitamins, and minerals, making it an essential part of your healthy ketogenic diet.

6 cups roughly chopped kale, tough ribs removed

1 garlic clove, very finely minced

Sea salt

Freshly ground black pepper

2 tablespoons extra-virgin olive oil

1 tablespoon white wine vinegar

1 large avocado, pitted, peeled, and diced

1. Place the kale in a large salad bowl. Add the garlic and season with salt and pepper. Drizzle with the olive oil.

2. Using your hands, massage the oil and garlic into the kale leaves until they become a darker shade of green and lose some of their liquid.

3. Sprinkle with the vinegar and toss gently to coat.

4. Gently fold in the diced avocado and serve immediately.

PER SERVING Calories: 188; Fat: 14g; Protein: 5g; Total Carbs: 15g; Fiber: 7g; Net Carbs: 8g
67% fat, 11% protein, 22% carbs

INGREDIENT TIP: To get the most flavor from the garlic, run the clove over a fine grater to produce a "purée," which will disperse more evenly over the salad.

Apple Cabbage Cumin Coleslaw

KETO
QUOTIENT
① 2 3

Serves 4 / Prep time: 5 minutes / Cook time: 0 minutes

DAIRY FREE • NUT FREE • VEGETARIAN • 30 MINUTES OR LESS

The combination of earthy cumin, sweet apples, and tangy mayonnaise makes this salad one you'll crave. It pairs well with barbecued dishes, especially the BBQ Baby Back Ribs (page 189).

¼ cup full-fat mayonnaise

½ teaspoon Dijon mustard

½ teaspoon ground cumin

Juice of 1 lemon

½ small head Savoy cabbage, shredded

½ red onion, thinly sliced

1 small Granny Smith apple, cored and cut into matchsticks

1. In a medium salad bowl, whisk together the mayonnaise, mustard, cumin, and lemon juice.

2. Add the cabbage and red onion, and using your hands, mix thoroughly. Fold in the apples and serve immediately.

PER SERVING Calories: 135; Fat: 10 g; Protein: 2g; Total Carbs: 11g; Fiber: 3g; Net Carbs: 8g 67% fat, 6% protein, 17% carbs

PREP TIP: To keep coleslaw from getting soggy, the solution is simple: Don't dress it until you're ready to serve it. Shredded more cabbage than you need? Only dress what you intend to eat.

Sesame Ginger Slaw

Serves 4 / Prep time: 10 minutes / Cook time: 0 minutes

DAIRY FREE • NUT FREE • VEGETARIAN • 30 MINUTES OR LESS

Soy ginger dressing is often loaded with sugar—as much as half of it may be brown sugar, honey, or even high-fructose corn syrup. Yikes! This version gets loads of flavor from fresh ginger and garlic, and a hint of sweetness from lime juice. If you want to sweeten it a little further, feel free to add a couple of drops of liquid stevia to the dressing.

2 tablespoons toasted sesame oil

2 tablespoons extra-virgin olive oil

2 tablespoons low-sodium soy sauce

1 tablespoon lime juice

1 teaspoon minced fresh ginger

1 teaspoon minced fresh garlic

Pinch red pepper flakes

½ small head Savoy cabbage, shredded

¼ cup roughly chopped cilantro

¼ cup roughly chopped mint

1 scallion, thinly sliced

4 tablespoons sesame seeds

1. In a medium salad bowl, whisk together the sesame oil, olive oil, soy sauce, lime juice, garlic, ginger, and red pepper flakes.

2. Add the cabbage, cilantro, mint, and scallion to the bowl and toss gently to mix. Sprinkle with the sesame seeds before serving.

PER SERVING Calories: 200; Fat: 19g; Protein: 4g; Total Carbs: 8g; Fiber: 4g; Net Carbs: 4g
86% fat, 8% protein, 6% carbs

INGREDIENT TIP: To improve the flavor of the sesame seeds, toast them in a dry skillet over medium heat for about 2 minutes until golden brown and fragrant.

Spinach Salad with Bacon and Soft-Boiled Eggs

Serves 4 / Prep time: 10 minutes / Cook time: 12 to 13 minutes

DAIRY FREE • NUT FREE • 30 MINUTES OR LESS

Bacon and eggs are a low-carb breakfast staple, but they're also delicious at lunch. Here they're paired with a generous helping of spinach. A 10-ounce package of fresh spinach may look like a lot, but once it is wilted, it shrinks dramatically.

4 eggs

5 ounces applewood smoked bacon, cut into pieces

2 tablespoons minced red onion or shallots

2 tablespoons extra-virgin olive oil

1 (10-ounce) package fresh spinach

1 teaspoon apple cider vinegar

Sea salt

Freshly ground black pepper

1. Place the whole eggs in a small saucepan and cover with fresh water. Bring to a simmer, remove from the heat and cover for 12 minutes. Remove the eggs to an ice-water bath and peel when cool enough to handle. Slice each of the eggs in half lengthwise.

2. Meanwhile, cook the bacon in a large skillet over medium-low heat until the bacon is crisp and has rendered most of its fat, about 10 minutes. Transfer it to a separate dish.

3. Add the olive oil and onion or shallots to the pan and cook for 2 to 3 minutes to soften.

4. Add the spinach to the pan and cook for about 1 minute, just until wilted but not yet losing its liquid. Sprinkle with the vinegar and season generously with salt and pepper.

5. Divide the spinach among the serving plates and top with equal amounts of the cooked bacon. Place two egg halves on top of each salad.

PER SERVING Calories: 352; Fat: 30g; Protein: 16g; Total Carbs: 4g; Fiber: 2g; Net Carbs: 2g
78% fat, 18% protein, 4% carbs

PREP TIP: Make a big batch of soft-boiled eggs ahead of time to use in this salad or enjoy for a snack. Mark the eggs gently with a pencil and store them in a separate egg carton.

Greek Salad with Shrimp

Serves 4 / Prep time: 10 minutes / Cook time: 0 minutes

NUT FREE • 30 MINUTES OR LESS

You can serve this classic Greek salad with any protein you prefer, but I like shrimp because it tastes great chilled, and I can throw the whole salad together in the morning and keep the dressing on the side until I'm ready to serve. It makes a great lunch or light dinner.

¼ cup extra-virgin olive oil

2 tablespoons white wine vinegar

1 teaspoon minced fresh thyme

1 teaspoon minced fresh oregano

1 teaspoon minced garlic

Sea salt

Freshly ground black pepper

8 cups roughly chopped
    romaine lettuce

1 small red onion, halved and
    thinly sliced

1 cup roughly chopped tomatoes

1 cup diced, peeled cucumber

½ cup pitted Kalamata olives

4 ounces feta cheese, crumbled

1 pound cooked shrimp,
    tails removed

1. In a small jar, combine the olive oil, vinegar, thyme, oregano, and garlic. Add salt and pepper. Cover tightly with a lid and shake vigorously.

2. In a large bowl, toss together the romaine lettuce, onion, tomatoes, cucumber, and olives. Pour the dressing over the salad and mix to coat thoroughly.

3. Divide the salad among the serving plates. Top with the feta cheese and cooked shrimp.

PER SERVING Calories: 382; Fat: 25g; Protein: 30g; Total Carbs: 9g; Fiber: 3g; Net Carbs: 6g
59% fat, 31% protein, 10% carbs

Essential Cobb Salad

Serves 4 / Prep time: 10 minutes / Cook time: 0 minutes

NUT FREE • 30 MINUTES OR LESS

Low-carb dieters tend to tire of endless bun-less cheeseburgers, so it's only fitting that Cobb salad be included in this book. This salad was created by Robert Cobb, who started a chain of restaurants that served hamburgers and hot dogs. He tired of the monotonous menu, and eventually tossed some lettuce, tomato, bacon, and cheese into a bowl with dressing, and the Cobb salad was born.

¼ cup extra-virgin olive oil

1 teaspoon Dijon mustard

2 tablespoons white wine vinegar

Sea salt

Freshly ground black pepper

8 cups roughly chopped butter or romaine lettuce

½ cup crumbled cooked bacon

2 eggs, hardboiled, peeled, and crumbled

¼ cup blue cheese crumbles

1 large avocado, pitted, peeled, and diced

1 small red onion, halved and thinly sliced

½ pint cherry tomatoes, halved

1. In a large salad bowl, whisk together the olive oil, mustard, and vinegar. Season with salt and pepper. Add the lettuce and toss gently to coat. Divide the salad among the serving bowls.

2. Top each salad with bacon, egg, blue cheese, avocado, red onion, and cherry tomatoes.

PER SERVING Calories: 500; Fat: 44g; Protein: 16g; Total Carbs: 11g; Fiber: 5g; Net Carbs: 6g 79% fat, 13% protein, 8% carbs

VARIATION TIP: For more protein, top each salad with 4 ounces of cooked chicken breast.

VARIATION PER SERVING Calories: 637; Fat: 47g; Protein: 42g; Total Carbs: 11g; Fiber: 5g; Net Carbs: 6g; 66% fat, 27% protein, 7% carbs

Spicy Serrano Gazpacho

Serves 4 / Prep time: 10 minutes / Cook time: 0 minutes

DAIRY FREE • NUT FREE • VEGETARIAN • 30 MINUTES OR LESS

The key to delicious gazpacho lies in using the absolute best tomatoes you can find. Heirloom tomatoes are a good choice and so are the locally grown tomatoes you can pick up at your farmers' market.

3 cups cored and diced vine-ripened
  tomatoes, divided
1 cucumber, peeled and
  diced, divided
1 serrano pepper, stem, seeds,
  and membranes removed,
  sliced in half

2 tablespoons red wine vinegar
¼ cup olive oil
Sea salt
Freshly ground black pepper
1 shallot, minced
2 tablespoons thinly sliced basil

1. In a blender, combine 1½ cups of the tomatoes, half of the cucumber, half of the pepper, the red wine vinegar, and the olive oil. Blend until smooth, and season with salt and pepper.

2. Taste the soup for spiciness level. If desired, add the remaining half of the pepper and blend again until smooth.

3. Stir in the remaining tomatoes, cucumber, shallot, and basil.

4. Chill for 30 minutes before serving.

PER SERVING Calories: 156; Fat: 14g; Protein: 2g; Total Carbs: 8g; Fiber: 2g; Net Carbs: 6g
81% fat, 5% protein, 14% carbs

VARIATION TIP: Make this soup a little more substantial by adding 2 tablespoons of crumbled feta cheese to each serving.

VARIATION PER SERVING Calories: 209; Fat: 18g; Protein: 4g; Total Carbs: 9g; Fiber: 2g; Net Carbs: 7g; 78% fat, 8% protein, 14% carbs

French Onion Soup

The traditional version of this soup is often topped with a slice of toast covered in melted cheese, which I have never quite understood. The bread becomes soggy and is such a disappointment. So, you're not missing much to leave it out! Instead, I like to serve this soup with Parmesan Crisps (page 72) on the side.

2 tablespoons butter

2 tablespoons olive oil

3 yellow onions, halved and
  thinly sliced

Pinch sea salt

¼ cup dry red wine

1 quart Beef Bone Broth (page 225)

1 sprig fresh thyme

1 sprig fresh rosemary

1. Heat a large pot over medium heat and melt the butter and olive oil. Add the onions and season with the salt. Cover and cook for 30 minutes.

2. Remove the lid and continue to cook until the onions are golden brown, about 30 more minutes. The longer they cook, the deeper the flavor becomes.

3. Pour in the red wine, broth, thyme, and rosemary. Bring to a simmer and cook for 20 minutes. Remove the herbs.

4. Allow to cool for 10 minutes before serving.

PER SERVING Calories: 185; Fat: 13g; Protein: 7g; Total Carbs: 9g; Fiber: 2g; Net Carbs: 7g
63% fat, 12% protein, 15% carbs

VARIATION TIP: To make this a full meal, add 1 pound of chicken thighs to the pan after the onion has caramelized and sear on each side for 2 minutes, before moving on to step 3.

VARIATION PER SERVING Calories: 333; Fat: 18g; Protein: 32g; Total Carbs: 9g; Fiber: 2g; Net Carbs: 7g; 49% fat, 38% protein, 13% carbs

Tomato Basil Soup

KETO
QUOTIENT

1 ② 3

Serves 4 / Prep time: 5 minutes / Cook time: 20 minutes

DAIRY FREE • NUT FREE • VEGETARIAN • 30 MINUTES OR LESS

I worked in an Italian restaurant in college, and this was one of our most popular soups. It's simple, but the olive oil and fresh basil make it so rich and flavorful.

¼ cup extra-virgin olive oil

1 cup diced onion

1 teaspoon minced garlic

1 (28-ounce) can whole plum
   tomatoes with basil

2 cups vegetable broth or Chicken
   Bone Broth (page 224)

¼ cup thinly sliced fresh basil

1. Heat the olive oil in a large pot over medium heat. Add the onion and garlic, and cook until soft and fragrant, about 10 minutes.

2. Pour the tomatoes and broth into the pot and simmer uncovered for 10 minutes.

3. Remove the soup from the heat. Use an immersion blender to purée the soup until very smooth. Alternatively, carefully transfer the soup in small batches to a blender and purée, allowing the heat to escape between pulses.

4. Stir in the fresh basil, and ladle the portions into soup bowls.

PER SERVING Calories: 167; Fat: 14g; Protein: 2g; Total Carbs: 11g; Fiber: 2g; Net Carbs: 9g
75% fat, 5% protein, 20% carbs

INGREDIENT TIP: You can purchase puréed tomatoes, but the flavor of whole plum tomatoes is substantially better, so just purée them yourself to get the best of both worlds.

VARIATION TIP: For an artful presentation, serve with additional fresh basil leaves and a few halved heirloom grape and cherry tomatoes along with a drizzle of olive oil.

Cream of Mushroom Soup

Serves 4 / Prep time: 10 minutes / Cook time: 20 minutes

NUT FREE • 30 MINUTES OR LESS

Discard every reference you have of cream of mushroom soup coming from a can. This version is not only more flavorful, but it's also free from the modified food starch and corn syrup used for thickening the canned variety.

6 tablespoons butter, divided

2 cups sliced mushrooms, divided

½ cup minced onions

1 teaspoon minced garlic

1 teaspoon minced thyme

2 tablespoons sherry (optional)

Sea salt

Freshly ground black pepper

1 quart hot Beef Bone Broth (page 225)

1 cup heavy cream

1. Heat 2 tablespoons of the butter in a large pot over medium-high heat. When the butter is very hot, add a generous handful of the mushrooms to the pot (about one-third of the total), making sure not to crowd the bottom of the pot. Brown the mushrooms, about 1 minute on each side.

2. Push the cooked mushrooms to the sides of the pot. Add another 2 tablespoons of butter and another generous handful of mushrooms. Brown and repeat with the remaining butter and mushrooms.

3. Turn the heat down to medium and add the onions, garlic, and thyme to the pan. Cook for 2 to 3 minutes, until the onions are beginning to soften, being careful not to burn the garlic.

4. Add the sherry (if using), and deglaze the pan with it by scraping up all of the browned bits from the bottom of the pan. Season with salt and pepper.

continued >

Cream of Mushroom Soup *continued*

5. Pour in the beef broth and simmer gently until the mushrooms are tender, about 8 minutes.

6. Stir in the heavy cream and cook over low heat until the soup is thick and velvety, about 2 minutes.

PER SERVING Calories: 335; Fat: 34g; Protein: 3g; Total Carbs: 6g; Fiber: 1g; Net Carbs: 5g
91% fat, 4% protein, 5% carbs

INGREDIENT TIP: It may sound like a hassle, but don't skip the process of browning the mushrooms in batches. When seared in butter, they give this soup a ton of flavor. Cooking them all at once yields too much liquid, so they stew instead of sear.

Chicken Marsala Soup

NUT FREE

 2 3

A few years ago, I wrote a cookbook devoted to soups, and this was one of my favorite recipes from the whole book. I've adapted this version to be lower in carbs, but it's still rich in all of the savory tastes of the original.

2 tablespoons extra-virgin olive oil

1 pound chicken thighs, cut into
   2-inch pieces

Sea salt

Freshly ground black pepper

1 onion, halved and thinly sliced

2 garlic cloves, smashed

4 tablespoons butter

2 cups cremini mushrooms,
   thinly sliced

½ cup Marsala wine

1½ quarts Beef Bone Broth (page 225)

1 sprig fresh rosemary

1. Place a large pot over medium-high heat and heat the olive oil. Season the chicken thighs with salt and pepper. Sear the chicken thighs until browned on both sides but not yet cooked through.

2. Transfer the chicken to a separate dish.

3. In the same pan, cook the onion and garlic until they begin to soften, about 5 minutes. Push them to the sides of the pan and melt the butter in the center.

4. Brown the mushrooms in two or three batches, pushing them to the side as you go. Season with salt and pepper.

5. Pour in the wine and beef stock, and add the rosemary. Return the chicken to the pot. Season with salt and pepper, cover, and simmer for 20 minutes.

PER SERVING Calories: 429; Fat: 26g; Protein: 38g; Total Carbs: 8g; Fiber: 1g; Net Carbs: 7g
55% fat, 35% protein, 7% carbs

Slow Cooker Pork Chile Verde

Serves 4 / Prep time: 5 minutes / Cook time: 8 hours

NUT FREE

As much as I love cooking—I do it for a living—there's something special about walking in the door after a long day and having dinner already prepared. This slow cooker supper is the perfect answer to busy week-nights. Creamy avocado and full-fat sour cream provide a cooling flavor contrast.

1 pound pork shoulder

1 yellow onion, halved and
   cut into thick slices

2 garlic cloves, smashed

1 (16-ounce) jar fire-roasted
   salsa verde

1 quart Chicken Bone Broth (page 224)

Sea salt

Freshly ground black pepper

1 small avocado, pitted, peeled, and
   thinly sliced

½ cup full-fat sour cream

1. Place the pork shoulder into a medium-size slow cooker and scatter the sliced onion and garlic over it. Season generously with salt and pepper.

2. Pour the salsa verde and chicken broth into the slow cooker, cover, and cook on low for 8 hours.

3. Shred the pork with two forks, and season with salt and pepper.

4. Serve with avocado and sour cream.

PER SERVING Calories: 496; Fat: 37g; Protein: 29g; Total Carbs: 11g; Fiber: 3g; Net Carbs: 8g
67% fat, 23% protein, 10% carbs

PREP TIP: To prepare this on the stove top, mix together all of the ingredients in a large pot over medium-high heat. Bring to a simmer, cover, and cook for 1½ hours, or until the pork easily shreds with a fork.

INGREDIENT TIP: For a more authentic version of this dish, use homemade salsa verde. On a rimmed baking sheet with 2 tablespoons of canola oil, spread out 1 pound of husked tomatillos, 1 onion cut into chunks, 4 unpeeled garlic cloves, and 2 Hatch chiles. Roast for 30 minutes at 375°F. Remove the peels from the garlic and chiles. In a blender, blend 2 tablespoons of lime juice and the roasted vegetables until mostly smooth.

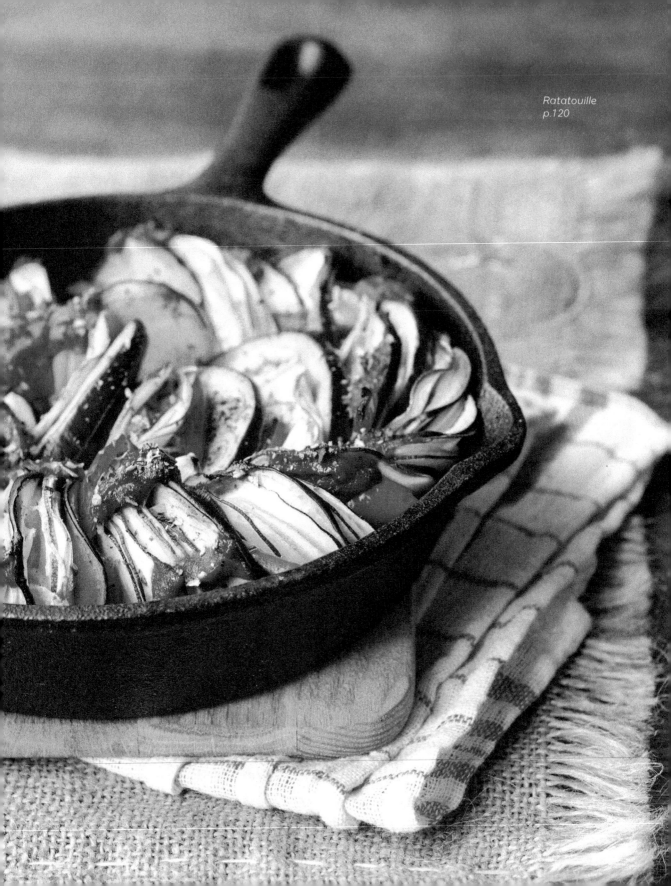

Ratatouille
p.120

CHAPTER SEVEN
Veggies & Sides

Radishes with Olive Mayo

Serves 1 / Prep time: 5 minutes / Cook time: 0 minutes

DAIRY FREE • NUT FREE • VEGETARIAN • 30 MINUTES OR LESS

The peppery bite of radishes provides the perfect contrast to this tangy, cool dip flecked with briny Kalamata olives. The recipe is simple, but to make it even easier, just serve the radishes with softened butter and sea salt, a classic combination.

4 medium radishes

2 tablespoons full-fat mayonnaise

1 tablespoon minced shallot
  or red onion

4 Kalamata olives, pitted and minced

⅛ teaspoon balsamic vinegar

1. Scrub the radishes and remove all but 1 inch of the leaves and stems. Pat the radishes dry with paper towels.

2. In a small bowl, whisk the mayonnaise, shallot, olives, and balsamic vinegar. Serve alongside the radishes as a dip.

PER SERVING Calories: 231; Fat: 24g; Protein: 0g; Total Carbs: 4g; Fiber: 1g; Net Carbs: 3g
94% fat, 0% protein, 6% carbs

INGREDIENT TIP: Remove the leaves immediately after you purchase radishes to prolong the shelf life of this root vegetable.

Quick Pickled Cucumbers

Serves 4 / Prep time: 5 minutes, plus 30 minutes to marinate / Cook time: 0 minutes

KETO
QUOTIENT

 2 3

DAIRY FREE • NUT FREE • VEGETARIAN • 30 MINUTES OR LESS

These cucumbers make a delicious low-carb, low-calorie side dish. I especially enjoy them with a tapas-style menu that includes cured meat, artisan cheese, and almonds.

1 English cucumber, cut into
  ½-inch pieces

¼ cup white wine vinegar

2 tablespoons minced fresh dill

1 teaspoon coriander seeds

¼ teaspoon red pepper flakes

¼ teaspoon sea salt

In a glass mixing bowl, toss together all of the ingredients. Cover and refrigerate for at least 30 minutes before serving.

PER SERVING Calories: 13; Fat: 0g; Protein: 1g; Total Carbs: 2g; Fiber: 1g; Net Carbs: 1g
0% fat, 23% protein, 67% carbs

VARIATION TIP: You can use blanched green beans in place of the cucumber if you'd like.

Mint-Marinated Artichoke Hearts

Serves 2 / Prep time: 5 minutes / Cook time: 0 minutes

DAIRY FREE • NUT FREE • VEGETARIAN • 30 MINUTES OR LESS

This is one of my favorite appetizers to snack on while I prepare a more substantial meal. I like to make it ahead of time and refrigerate it for several hours until I'm ready to serve it to allow the mint, garlic, and lemon to infuse the marinade with flavor.

1 cup drained jarred artichoke hearts

2 tablespoons extra-virgin olive oil

1 tablespoon minced fresh mint

Zest and juice of 1 lemon

1 garlic clove, finely minced

Sea salt

Freshly ground black pepper

In a small bowl, toss together the artichoke hearts, olive oil, mint, lemon zest and juice, and garlic. Season with salt and pepper. Serve immediately, or cover and refrigerate until ready to serve.

PER SERVING Calories: 212; Fat: 20g; Protein: 1g; Total Carbs: 9g; Fiber: 2g; Net Carbs: 7g
85% fat, 1% protein, 14% carbs

VARIATION TIP: If you don't care for mint, swap it for a teaspoon each of fresh thyme, parsley, and oregano.

Pesto Sautéed Vegetables

Serves 4 / Prep time: 5 minutes / Cook time: 5 minutes

VEGETARIAN • 30 MINUTES OR LESS

Pesto elevates simple sautéed vegetables from everyday food to something I look forward to all day. Prepare all of the ingredients ahead of time because the cooking goes really quickly once you get started.

2 tablespoons canola oil

1 yellow or orange bell pepper, seeds and ribs removed, thinly sliced

1 medium zucchini, cut into ½-inch pieces

1 cup grape tomatoes

½ cup Pesto (page 223)

Sea salt

Freshly ground black pepper

1. Heat a large skillet over high heat. When the skillet is hot, add the canola oil, tilting the pan to coat. Allow the oil to get hot.

2. Add the pepper and zucchini to the skillet, and sauté for 3 minutes until the vegetables are beginning to brown. Add the tomatoes and cook until hot but not bursting, about 2 minutes.

3. Remove the pan from the heat and add the pesto. Stir to coat the vegetables in the pesto, and season with salt and pepper.

PER SERVING Calories: 239; Fat: 21g; Protein: 3g; Total Carbs: 9g; Fiber: 2g; Net Carbs: 7g
79% fat, 6% protein, 15% carbs

INGREDIENT TIP: Although the term "sauté" is often mistakenly applied to cooking anything in a pan, it actually means to cook something over high heat in oil. Sautéing is especially important for preparing zucchini because it keeps the vegetable crisp and tender.

Pan-Roasted Brussels Sprouts with Bacon

Serves 4 / Prep time: 5 minutes / Cook time: 12 to 13 minutes

DAIRY FREE • NUT FREE • 30 MINUTES OR LESS

This simple recipe has popped up on appetizer menus around the country, winning people over to the leafy green's best features. I tried it recently at a tapas restaurant where the Brussels sprouts had first been shredded and loved it!

4 applewood smoked bacon slices, cut into pieces

1 pound Brussels sprouts, wilted outer leaves and tough stem ends removed

Sea salt

Freshly ground black pepper

1 tablespoon sherry vinegar or apple cider vinegar

1. Cook the bacon in a large skillet over medium-low heat until the bacon renders all of its fat and begins to crisp. Transfer the bacon to a separate dish with a slotted spoon.

2. While the bacon is cooking, run the Brussels sprouts through the shredder of a food processor to form long, thin shreds.

3. Increase the heat to medium-high. Cook the shredded Brussels sprouts in the bacon fat for 2 to 3 minutes, until just wilted. Season with salt and pepper, and drizzle with the vinegar just before serving. Top each serving with the cooked bacon pieces.

PER SERVING Calories: 210; Fat: 16g; Protein: 10g; Total Carbs: 9g; Fiber: 3g; Net Carbs: 6g
69% fat, 17% protein, 14% carbs

Bacon-Wrapped Asparagus Bundles

Serves 4 / Prep time: 5 minutes / Cook time: 15 to 17 minutes

DAIRY FREE • NUT FREE • 30 MINUTES OR LESS

KETO
QUOTIENT

1 ② 3

If you don't think you're a fan of asparagus, or any vegetable for that matter, roast it in the oven until browned on the outside and tender on the inside. Of course, wrapping it in bacon doesn't hurt either.

1 bunch asparagus, ends trimmed

2 tablespoons extra-virgin olive oil

Sea salt

Freshly ground black pepper

8 slices bacon

1. Preheat the oven to 375°F. Line a baking sheet with parchment paper.

2. Coat the asparagus in the olive oil and season generously with salt and pepper.

3. Place 3 to 4 asparagus spears over a slice of bacon and roll the meat around to hold the asparagus together. Place it on the baking sheet. Repeat with the remaining asparagus and bacon.

4. Bake for 15 to 17 minutes, or until the asparagus is wilted and the bacon is crispy.

PER SERVING (2 bundles) Calories: 202; Fat: 17g; Protein: 10g; Total Carbs: 4g; Fiber: 2g; Net Carbs: 3g; 76% fat, 20% protein, 4% carbs

INGREDIENT TIP: Use thin-cut bacon for best results. It cooks at a similar rate to the asparagus and renders all of its fat, so the asparagus is coated in delicious bacon drippings and the bacon is crisp.

Roasted Cauliflower with Parsley and Pine Nuts

Serves 4 / Prep time: 5 minutes / Cook time: 30 minutes

DAIRY FREE • VEGETARIAN • 30 MINUTES OR LESS

This appetizer is a staple in my house. It's loaded with flavor and is a healthy alternative to fries or potato chips. You can use this method to roast other vegetables, such as eggplant, red cabbage, onions, asparagus, or carrots.

1 small head cauliflower,
    broken into small florets
4 cloves garlic, minced
Zest and juice of 1 lemon
¼ cup olive oil

Sea salt
Freshly ground black pepper
¼ cup roughly chopped fresh parsley
¼ cup roughly chopped toasted
    pine nuts

1. Preheat the oven to 400°F.

2. Spread the cauliflower out on a rimmed baking sheet and add the garlic, lemon zest, and olive oil. Toss to coat, trying to keep the garlic on the cauliflower and not just on the pan. Season with salt and pepper.

3. Roast for 30 minutes, or until the cauliflower is deeply browned on the bottom and soft. Toss with the lemon juice, parsley, and pine nuts before serving.

PER SERVING Calories: 192; Fat: 18g; Protein: 2g; Total Carbs: 7g; Fiber: 3g; Net Carbs: 4g
84% fat, 4% protein, 12% carbs

Grilled Balsamic Cabbage

Serves 4 / Prep time: 10 minutes / Cook time: 17 to 19 minutes

DAIRY FREE • NUT FREE • VEGETARIAN • 30 MINUTES OR LESS

Char-grilling red cabbage is a great way to change up your veggie game. The ends become crispy and blackened while the thicker leaves are tender and succulent. Take the party inside if you must and prepare the recipe in the oven.

1 small head red cabbage

¼ cup extra-virgin olive oil

2 tablespoons balsamic vinegar

1 teaspoon Dijon mustard

¼ teaspoon ground cumin

½ teaspoon sea salt

¼ teaspoon freshly ground black pepper

1. Preheat a gas or charcoal grill to medium-high.

2. Slice the cabbage into 16 wedges.

3. In a small jar, combine the olive oil, balsamic vinegar, mustard, cumin, salt, and pepper. Cover tightly with a lid and shake vigorously.

4. Cut 16 small squares of aluminum foil. Place a cabbage wedge onto a square of foil and drizzle with about 1 teaspoon of the balsamic mixture. Fold the foil into a tight package. Repeat with the remaining cabbage.

5. Place the foil packets onto the grill grate and cook for 12 to 15 minutes, until the cabbage is tender. Remove the cabbage from the foil and carefully place them directly onto the grill. Grill on each side for about 2 minutes, just enough to infuse it with the smoky flavor and get it a bit crunchy.

PER SERVING Calories: 169; Fat: 14g; Protein: 3g; Total Carbs: 11g; Fiber: 4g; Net Carbs: 7g
75% fat, 7% protein, 18% carbs

PREP TIP: To prepare this dish in the oven, coat the cabbage with the dressing and roast uncovered for 25 to 30 minutes at 375°F, until the cabbage is tender and crisp around the edges.

Celery Root Purée

Serves 4 / Prep time: 10 minutes / Cook time: 30 minutes

NUT FREE • VEGETARIAN

Celeriac, also called celery root, has less than half the carbs of potatoes. It has a faint celery taste, which is complemented by onion and garlic. Heavy cream makes it absolutely luxurious. You may never go back to mashed potatoes again.

4 cups peeled, diced celeriac

½ cup diced onion

1 garlic clove, minced

1 sprig fresh thyme

1 cup vegetable broth or Chicken
   Bone Broth (page 224)

1 cup heavy cream

Sea salt

2 tablespoons butter

1. Place the celeriac, onion, garlic, thyme, broth, and cream in a large pot. Season generously with salt. Bring to a simmer over medium-low heat. Cover and cook for 30 minutes, until the celeriac is tender.

2. Discard the thyme sprig.

3. Strain the vegetables and transfer to a food processor, reserving the cooking liquid. Purée until smooth, adding some cooking liquid as needed to reach the desired consistency. Stir in the butter.

PER SERVING Calories: 307; Fat: 28g; Protein: 3g; Total Carbs: 13g; Fiber: 2g; Net Carbs: 11g
82% fat, 3% protein, 15% carbs

PREP TIP: To remove the tough, knobby skin from the celery root, cut off each end with a chef's knife. Stand it on one end and use the knife to shave away the exterior pieces.

Smoky Stewed Kale

Serves 4 / Prep time: 5 minutes / Cook time: 30 minutes

KETO
QUOTIENT

1 ② 3

DAIRY FREE • NUT FREE • VEGETARIAN

I thought I only loved raw kale—until I tried this stewed kale and instantly fell in love with it. The texture is tender and barely chewy. The flavor is tangy with a hint of smokiness. For a vegetarian version, choose the vegetable broth. I personally prefer the flavor that the Chicken Bone Broth imparts.

¼ cup extra-virgin olive oil

½ cup minced onion

2 garlic cloves, minced

Pinch red pepper flakes

1 teaspoon smoked paprika

1 tablespoon tomato paste

6 cups roughly chopped kale

½ cup vegetable broth or Chicken Bone Broth (page 224)

1 tablespoon red wine vinegar

1. Heat the olive oil in a large skillet over medium heat. Cook the onion and garlic until they begin to soften, about 5 minutes. Add the red pepper flakes, paprika, and tomato paste, and cook until the onion and garlic begin to caramelize.

2. Add the kale, broth, and red wine vinegar to the skillet, and cook for 20 to 25 minutes, stirring often, until the kale is tender and most of the liquid has evaporated.

PER SERVING Calories: 190; Fat: 15g; Protein: 5g; Total Carbs: 14g; Fiber: 5g; Net Carbs: 9g
71% fat, 11% protein, 18% carbs

INGREDIENT TIP: To ensure the kale leaves and stems cook at about the same rate, roughly chop the leaves and finely dice the stems.

Creamed Broccoli

Serves 4 / Prep time: 5 minutes / Cook time: 16 minutes

NUT FREE • 30 MINUTES OR LESS

This creamy vegetable side dish is my idea of comfort food. Serve with a perfectly seared steak for a complete low-carb meal.

1 tablespoon olive oil

2 garlic cloves, minced

Pinch red pepper flakes

1 bunch broccoli, broken into florets,
   stems chopped

½ cup Chicken Bone Broth (page 224)
   or low-sodium chicken broth

Sea salt

½ cup heavy cream

1. In a large skillet with a lid, heat the olive oil over medium heat. Add the garlic and red pepper flakes. Cook for about 1 minute, just until fragrant.

2. Add the broccoli and broth. Season with salt. Cover the skillet, and cook until the broccoli is tender, about 15 minutes.

3. Remove the lid, and stir in the heavy cream. Use an immersion blender or a potato masher to break up the broccoli. It should be partially smooth with some chunks remaining.

PER SERVING Calories: 202; Fat: 17g; Protein: 8g; Total Carbs: 10g; Fiber: 5g; Net Carbs: 5g
76% fat, 16% protein, 8% carbs

Stuffed Mushrooms

Serves 4 / Prep time: 10 minutes / Cook time: 20 to 25 minutes

KETO
QUOTIENT

1 2 ③

NUT FREE • VEGETARIAN

I often make an entire meal of nothing but appetizers because I love sampling many different foods at once. Mushrooms are a great low-carb vegetable, and these stuffed mushrooms are loaded with flavor.

12 cremini mushrooms,
   stems removed

6 ounces cream cheese

¼ cup Parmesan cheese

2 garlic cloves, minced

2 teaspoons minced fresh thyme

Sea salt

Freshly ground black pepper

1. Preheat the oven to 400°F.

2. Line a baking sheet with parchment paper. Place the mushrooms cap-side down on the baking sheet.

3. In a small mixing bowl, mix together the cream cheese, Parmesan cheese, garlic, and thyme. Season with salt and pepper.

4. Divide the mixture among the mushroom caps.

5. Bake for 20 to 25 minutes, or until the mushrooms are soft and the tops are golden brown. Allow to rest for 5 minutes before serving.

PER SERVING Calories: 186; Fat: 17g; Protein: 7g; Total Carbs: 4g; Fiber: 1g; Net Carbs: 3g
81% fat, 14% protein, 5% carbs

Ratatouille

Serves 4 / Prep time: 10 minutes / Cook time: 1½ hours

DAIRY FREE • NUT FREE • VEGETARIAN

This simple Provençal vegetable dish is so much more than the sum of its parts. Eggplant, zucchini, and plum tomatoes are roasted in a generous amount of olive oil and a splash of balsamic vinegar until they're meltingly tender and then topped with fresh basil. This dish tastes even better the next day, so double the recipe and plan for leftovers.

½ cup canned plum tomatoes and juices, divided

½ cup extra-virgin olive oil, divided

1 Japanese eggplant, thinly sliced

1 zucchini, thinly sliced

4 Roma tomatoes, thinly sliced

2 garlic cloves, minced

1 teaspoon minced thyme

Sea salt

Freshly ground black pepper

1 tablespoon balsamic vinegar

¼ cup roughly chopped fresh basil

1. Hand crush the plum tomatoes and spread half of the mixture into the bottom of a baking dish. Pour in ¼ cup of the olive oil.

2. Place the eggplant, zucchini, and tomato slices in the dish in a circular pattern, alternating between the ingredients.

3. Sprinkle the garlic, thyme, and remaining plum tomatoes over the vegetables. Season generously with salt and pepper.

4. Drizzle the remaining olive oil over the vegetables. Cover the dish with parchment paper or foil and bake for 1 hour.

5. Remove the foil and drizzle the balsamic vinegar over the vegetables. Bake uncovered for another 30 minutes, or until the vegetables are very tender and most of the liquid has evaporated from the dish. Serve warm, garnished with the basil.

PER SERVING Calories: 292; Fat: 27g; Protein: 2g; Total Carbs: 12g; Fiber: 4g; Net Carbs: 8g
83% fat, 5% protein, 16% carbs

VARIATION TIP: For more color, swap the second zucchini with a yellow summer squash.

Caramelized Fennel

Serves 4 / Prep time: 5 minutes / Cook time: 30 minutes

DAIRY FREE • NUT FREE • VEGETARIAN

Once you try oven-roasted caramelized fennel, it may become your new favorite vegetable. It becomes tender, chewy, and beautifully caramelized.

2 fennel bulbs

¼ cup extra-virgin olive oil

Sea salt

Freshly ground black pepper

1. Preheat the oven to 375°F.

2. Remove the fennel stems and fronds. Cut the fennel bulbs into 8 to 12 wedges, keeping the root ends intact.

3. Spread the fennel on a rimmed baking sheet. Drizzle with the olive oil and turn over to coat. Season with salt and pepper.

4. Roast for 30 minutes, or until the fennel is tender and gently browned on the bottom.

PER SERVING Calories: 156; Fat: 14g; Protein: 2g; Total Carbs: 9g; Fiber: 4g; Net Carbs: 5g 79% fat, 1% protein, 20% carbs

VARIATION TIP: Add 1 thinly sliced orange to the pan while roasting the fennel. It becomes chewy and sweet from being roasted and adds only 1.5 grams of net carbs to each serving.

Sautéed Zucchini with Mint and Pine Nuts

Serves 4 / Prep time: 5 minutes / Cook time: 7 minutes

DAIRY FREE • VEGETARIAN • 30 MINUTES OR LESS

This dish is perfect in the summertime when mint and zucchini abound. If I have them in my pantry, I also like to use preserved lemons in place of the lemon zest, but this isn't essential for great taste.

¼ cup pine nuts

2 tablespoons canola oil

2 medium zucchini, cut into
 ½-inch pieces

2 garlic cloves, minced

Zest and juice of 1 lemon

2 tablespoons minced mint

Sea salt

Freshly ground black pepper

1. Heat a large skillet over high heat. Toast the pine nuts until fragrant and beginning to brown, 1 to 2 minutes.

2. Transfer the pine nuts to a cutting board, and chop roughly.

3. Add the canola oil to the same skillet, tilting to coat. When the canola oil is heated, add the zucchini. Sauté for 5 minutes until the zucchini is well browned.

4. Remove the skillet from the heat. Add the garlic, lemon zest and juice, mint, and chopped pine nuts, and toss to mix. Season with salt and pepper.

PER SERVING Calories: 125; Fat: 11g; Protein: 2g; Total Carbs: 6g; Fiber: 2g; Net Carbs: 4g
79% fat, 6% protein, 15% carbs

VARIATION TIP: Instead of sautéing the zucchini, cut them into long spears, coat them in the canola oil, and place them on a hot grill. Remove them from the grill while they still have some crisp and chop them into ½-inch dice. Toss with the garlic, lemon zest and juice, mint, and pine nuts.

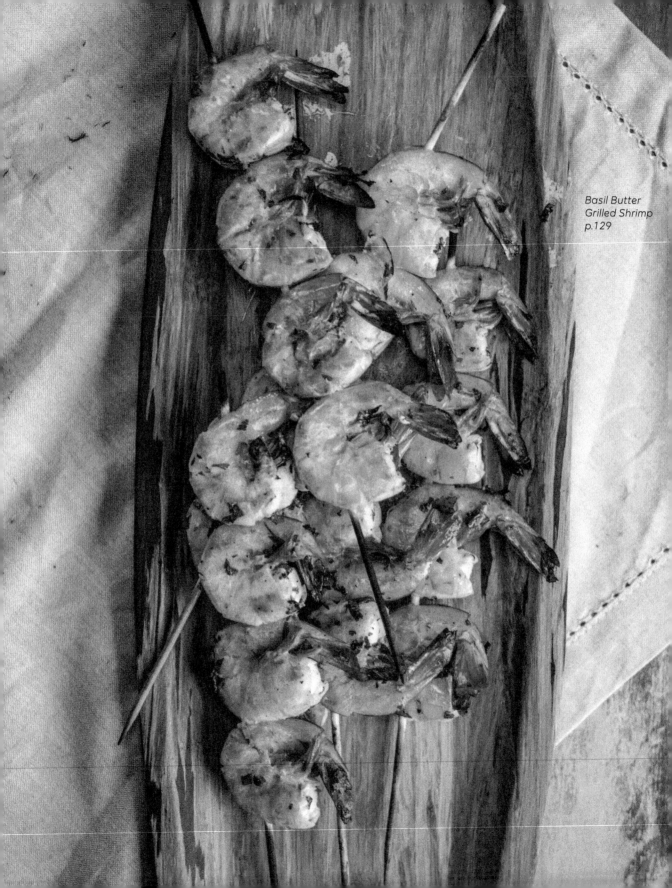

*Basil Butter
Grilled Shrimp
p.129*

CHAPTER EIGHT
Fish & Seafood

Pan-Seared Butter Scallops

Serves 4 / Prep time: 5 minutes / Cook time: 5 minutes

NUT FREE • 30 MINUTES OR LESS

Scallops cooked over high heat and basted with butter and garlic are just about as good as it gets for me. The texture of the scallops is similar to that of lobster, and they cost less, though they are still somewhat pricey. Splurge on extra-large diver scallops or sea scallops if you can. Prepare the Sautéed Zucchini with Mint and Pine Nuts (page 123) in the same pan for a complete meal.

4 tablespoons butter

2 tablespoons extra-virgin olive oil

1 pound large scallops

Sea salt

Freshly ground black pepper

2 teaspoons roughly chopped garlic

¼ cup roughly chopped fresh parsley

1. Heat a large skillet over high heat. Melt the butter and add the olive oil.

2. Pat the scallops dry with paper towels and season generously with salt and pepper.

3. When the butter and oil are hot, place the scallops in the pan, being sure not to crowd them.

4. Tilt the pan slightly and pick up a spoonful of the melted butter. Drizzle this over the scallops as they cook. Sear for about 2 minutes on the first side. Carefully flip and sear on the second side for 2 more minutes, or until the scallops are cooked through and opaque in the center.

5. During the last minute of cooking, add the garlic and parsley, and spoon the flavored oil and butter over the scallops.

PER SERVING Calories: 324; Fat: 21g; Protein: 29g; Total Carbs: 5g; Fiber: 1g; Net Carbs: 4g 59% fat, 36% protein, 5% carbs

Mussels with Lemon and Thyme

Serves 4 / Prep time: 10 minutes / Cook time: 18 to 20 minutes

NUT FREE • 30 MINUTES OR LESS

One of the first techniques I learned in classical French cooking was whisking cold butter into reduced wine. The acids in the wine act on the milk solids in the butter to produce a thick, luxurious, and tangy sauce that will have you licking the pot clean. Serve these mussels with steamed green beans or a few pieces of Cloud Bread (page 216).

2 tablespoons extra-virgin olive oil

1 medium onion, halved and
    thinly sliced

4 garlic cloves, smashed

2 sprigs fresh thyme

½ cup dry white wine

½ cup Chicken Bone Broth (page 224)
    or low-sodium chicken broth

2 pounds fresh mussels, scrubbed
    and de-bearded

Sea salt

Freshly ground black pepper

4 tablespoons cold butter,
    cut into pieces

¼ cup roughly chopped fresh parsley

1 lemon, cut into wedges

1. Heat the olive oil in a large pot over medium heat. Cook the onion for 7 to 8 minutes, until it begins to soften.

2. Add the garlic and thyme and cook for 30 seconds.

3. Add the wine and cook for 2 minutes to burn off some of the alcohol.

4. Add the chicken broth and the mussels to the pot. Season with salt and pepper. Toss well.

5. Cover and steam for 8 to 10 minutes, until all of the mussels have opened. Discard any that have not opened after 10 minutes. Remove the cooked mussels to a serving dish.

6. Return the pot to the heat and simmer the cooking liquid until reduced to about ⅓ cup.

continued >

7. Remove the pot from the heat and whisk in the butter 1 tablespoon at a time. It will thicken as the butter is added.

8. Pour the sauce over the mussels and sprinkle with the fresh parsley. Serve with lemon wedges.

PER SERVING Calories: 388; Fat: 26g; Protein: 28g; Total Carbs: 11g; Fiber: 1g; Net Carbs: 10g 60% fat, 30% protein, 10% carbs

INGREDIENT TIP: Scrub and remove the beards from the mussels just prior to cooking them. Discard any broken mussels as well as any that are already open and don't immediately shut when gently tapped.

Basil Butter Grilled Shrimp

Serves 4 / Prep time: 10 minutes / Cook time: 5 minutes

NUT FREE • 30 MINUTES OR LESS

KETO
QUOTIENT

1 ② 3

Fresh basil and lime juice make these shrimp juicy and flavorful. They are bursting with the flavors of summer. But if you want to prepare them in the dead of winter, pop them onto a broiler pan and cook them in the oven under a hot broiler for 2 to 3 minutes. Serve with Cucumber, Tomato, and Avocado Salad (page 88) for a complete meal.

½ cup butter, at room temperature

½ cup roughly chopped fresh basil

Zest and juice of 1 lime

1 pound large EZ-peel shrimp

1. In a small mixing bowl, mix together the butter, basil, and lime zest.

2. Spoon the butter mixture into each shrimp between the meat and the shell.

3. Thread the shrimp onto four bamboo skewers, about four shrimp per skewer. Place them on a hot grill and cook for 1 to 2 minutes per side, until gently charred.

PER SERVING Calories: 328; Fat: 25g; Protein: 23g; Total Carbs: 2g; Fiber: 0g; Net Carbs: 2g
70% fat, 28% protein, 2% carbs

PREP TIP: To keep all of the delicious basil butter from dripping into the grill, take care not to let the peels slip off the shrimp while grilling.

Fish Veracruz

Serves 4 / Prep time: 10 minutes / Cook time: 22 minutes

NUT FREE • 30 MINUTES OR LESS

The briny flavors of capers and olives blend into the spicy, sweet stewed tomatoes in this delicious fish dish. Whisking butter into the sauce makes it especially rich and delicious. Serve with Cauliflower Rice (page 218) for a complete meal.

¼ cup extra-virgin olive oil

¼ cup diced yellow onion

2 teaspoons roughly chopped garlic

Pinch red pepper flakes

2 tablespoons minced fresh parsley

1 teaspoon minced oregano

¼ cup pitted green olives

2 tablespoons drained capers

1 cup canned plum tomatoes with juices, hand crushed

1 tablespoon red wine vinegar

1¼ pounds red snapper, cut into 4 (5-ounce) fillets

3 tablespoons cold butter, cut into pieces

Sea salt

Freshly ground black pepper

1. Heat the olive oil in a large skillet over medium heat. Cook the onion, garlic, and red pepper flakes until beginning to soften, about 5 minutes. Add the parsley, oregano, olives, capers, tomatoes, and vinegar to the skillet and cook for 10 minutes, until the sauce has reduced somewhat and the tomatoes are pulpy.

2. Season the fish generously on both sides with salt and pepper, then add the fillets to the pan, spooning some of the sauce over the fish. Cook for about 3 minutes on each side, or until the fish flakes easily with a fork.

3. Transfer the cooked fish to a serving platter.

4. Remove the pan from the heat and whisk the cold butter into the tomato mixture one tablespoon at a time. Pour the sauce over the cooked fish and serve immediately.

PER SERVING Calories: 434; Fat: 27g; Protein: 38g; Total Carbs: 8g; Fiber: 2g; Net Carbs: 6g
58% fat, 35% protein, 7% carbs

INGREDIENT TIP: Any firm white fish can be used in this recipe. Try tilapia in place of the snapper.

Chimichurri Shrimp

Serves 4 / Prep time: 10 minutes / Cook time: 2 to 3 minutes

DAIRY FREE • NUT FREE • 30 MINUTES OR LESS

Chimichurri is an Argentinian condiment that can be used on grilled meat, fish, or anywhere you're looking for loads of flavor and low carbs. Traditionally the sauce is made with parsley, but I like the addition of cilantro. Choose whatever option suits your palate.

½ cup plus 1 tablespoon extra-virgin olive oil, divided

½ cup roughly chopped parsley

½ cup roughly chopped cilantro

1 tablespoon fresh oregano

3 garlic cloves, smashed

1 shallot, peeled and diced

½ teaspoon sea salt

¼ teaspoon red pepper flakes

2 tablespoons red wine vinegar

1½ pounds large shrimp, peeled and deveined

1. In a blender, pulse ½ cup of the olive oil, parsley, cilantro, oregano, garlic, shallot, sea salt, and red pepper flakes until nearly smooth. Stir in the red wine vinegar.

2. Heat the remaining tablespoon of olive oil in a large skillet over medium-high heat. Sauté the shrimp for 2 to 3 minutes, or until barely cooked through. Pour the chimichurri sauce into the pan to briefly warm it for about 30 seconds, and then remove from the heat.

PER SERVING Calories: 459; Fat: 33g; Protein: 35g; Total Carbs: 4g; Fiber: 1g; Net Carbs: 3g
65% fat, 31% protein, 4% carbs

PREP TIP: If you want to make the chimichurri sauce ahead of time, wait to add the salt and vinegar until just before serving.

Pepper-Crusted Salmon
with Wilted Kale

Serves 4 / Prep time: 5 minutes / Cook time: 5 minutes

DAIRY FREE • 30 MINUTES OR LESS

Growing up in the Pacific Northwest, I fell in love with salmon and its rich, creamy texture. Blueberries and hazelnuts are also Northwest favorites, so I've added them to this dish, but feel free to improvise and use any nuts and dark berries you have on hand or skip them altogether.

1½ pounds salmon, cut into
    4 (6-ounce) fillets
2 tablespoons coconut oil, melted
1 tablespoon freshly ground
    black pepper
½ teaspoon coarse sea salt, divided

1 bunch Lacinato kale, tough ribs
    removed and roughly chopped
2 tablespoons extra-virgin olive oil
1 teaspoon red wine vinegar
¼ cup roughly chopped hazelnuts
½ cup fresh blueberries (optional)

1. Preheat a large skillet over medium-high heat.

2. Coat the salmon fillets with the oil and then season liberally with the pepper and salt.

3. In the hot skillet, sear the salmon for about 2 minutes on each side, until it flakes easily with a fork but is still a deeper shade of pink on the inside. It will continue to cook for a few minutes after it has been removed from the pan.

4. While the salmon is cooking, place the kale in a large bowl, season with a generous pinch of sea salt, and drizzle with the olive oil. Using your hands, massage the oil and salt into the kale until it releases some of its liquid and becomes soft. Season with the red wine vinegar. Divide the kale among the serving plates and top with equal amounts of the hazelnuts and blueberries (if using).

continued >

5. Serve the salmon fillets alongside the kale.

PER SERVING Calories: 442; Fat: 29g; Protein: 37g; Total Carbs: 8g; Fiber: 3g; Net Carbs: 5g
60% fat, 33% protein, 7% carbs

INGREDIENT TIP: I prefer the bubbled texture of Lacinato kale in this recipe, but if you can't get it, other varieties of kale will work just as well.

Halibut in Tomato Basil Sauce

Serves 4 / Prep time: 10 minutes / Cook time: 20 minutes

DAIRY FREE • NUT FREE • 30 MINUTES OR LESS

A friend of mine is into spear fishing and landed an enormous halibut off the coast of Santa Barbara. He generously shared his catch with us and even offered to cook it. Whether you score your fish from the ocean or the frozen section of the grocery store, serve it with this simple tomato basil sauce, which balances the meaty texture of halibut with bright acidity and fragrant herbs.

8 tablespoons extra-virgin olive oil, divided

2 large garlic cloves, minced

1 pint grape tomatoes, halved

¼ cup dry white wine

Juice of 1 lemon

½ cup roughly chopped fresh basil

Sea salt

Freshly ground black pepper

1¼ pounds halibut, cut into 4 (5-ounce) fillets

1. Heat 6 tablespoons of the olive oil in a small saucepan over medium heat. Cook the garlic for about 30 seconds, until fragrant.

2. Add the tomatoes and cook for 10 minutes, until they partially break down. Stir in the wine and simmer for 1 to 2 minutes to cook off the alcohol.

3. Stir in the basil and lemon juice and season generously with salt and pepper.

4. While the sauce is cooking, heat the remaining 2 tablespoons of olive oil in a large skillet over medium-high heat. Season the halibut fillets liberally with salt and pepper. Sear on each side for 3 to 4 minutes, or until the fish flakes easily with a fork.

PER SERVING Calories: 467; Fat: 31g; Protein: 38g; Total Carbs: 5g; Fiber: 0g; Net Carbs: 5g
60% fat, 33% protein, 7% carbs

SUBSTITUTION TIP: Halibut can be a bit pricey, so you can swap it for cod if you wish—the nutrition information is roughly the same. Cod cooks more quickly, so reduce the cooking time to 2 to 3 minutes per side.

Macadamia-Crusted Halibut with Mango Coulis

Serves 4 / Prep time: 10 minutes / Cook time: 10 minutes

DAIRY FREE • 30 MINUTES OR LESS

I know what you're thinking: How could mango ever appear in a low-carb cookbook? It's true, the fruit does contain a fair bit of natural sugar if you eat the whole thing in one sitting. But when judiciously portioned and blended with coconut milk and lime juice, it only adds a mere 2 grams of net carbs per serving. Worth it!

½ cup finely chopped
  macadamia nuts

½ teaspoon sea salt

¼ teaspoon freshly ground
  black pepper

¼ teaspoon garlic powder

½ teaspoon onion powder

1¼ pounds halibut, cut into
  4 (5-ounce) fillets

2 tablespoons coconut oil

½ cup diced mango

1 tablespoon lime juice

½ cup full-fat coconut milk

4 sprigs fresh cilantro, for garnish

1. Preheat the oven to 425°F. Line a rimmed baking sheet with parchment paper.

2. In a shallow dish, mix together the macadamia nuts, salt, pepper, garlic powder, and onion powder.

3. Coat the halibut fillets in the coconut oil and then dredge in the nut mixture. Place the fillets onto the baking sheet, and bake for 12 minutes, or until the fish flakes easily with a fork.

4. While the halibut is cooking, in a blender, purée the mango, lime juice, and coconut milk until very smooth.

5. Drizzle a few tablespoons of the mango coulis over each plate and then top with the baked halibut and a sprig of cilantro.

PER SERVING Calories: 423; Fat: 27g; Protein: 40g; Total Carbs: 6g; Fiber: 2g; Net Carbs: 4g 57% fat, 38% protein, 5% carbs

VARIATION TIP: If you prefer a savory sauce, swap out the mango in step 4 for 1 tablespoon of shallots and ¼ cup of roughly chopped mint. Season with salt before serving.

VARIATION PER SERVING Calories: 412; Fat: 27g; Protein: 40g; Total Carbs: 4g; Fiber: 2g; Net Carbs: 2g; 58% fat, 39% protein, 3% carbs

Moroccan Salmon
with Cauliflower Rice Pilaf

Serves 4 / Prep time: 5 minutes / Cook time: 10 minutes

DAIRY FREE • 30 MINUTES OR LESS

The spice blend in this recipe brings a hint of the Mediterranean to this dish. Preserved lemons are commonly used in Moroccan cooking and are one of my favorite pantry staples, but you can use a teaspoon of lemon zest if you don't have them.

1 medium head of cauliflower, broken into florets

3 tablespoons coconut oil, melted, divided

1 tablespoon extra-virgin olive oil

1 teaspoon white wine vinegar

1 tablespoon minced preserved lemons (optional)

¼ cup roughly chopped mint

¼ cup roughly chopped pistachios

½ teaspoon coarse sea salt, plus more for seasoning pilaf, divided

Freshly ground black pepper

1¼ pounds salmon, cut into 4 (5-ounce) fillets

1 teaspoon ground cumin

1 teaspoon ground coriander

1 teaspoon ground ginger

1 teaspoon paprika

1. Pulse cauliflower in a food processor until coarsely ground, about the size and texture of rice.

2. Squeeze the cauliflower by the handful over the sink to remove excess moisture.

3. Heat 1 tablespoon of the coconut oil in a large skillet over medium-high heat. Stir-fry the cauliflower for 5 minutes, until just heated through.

4. Sprinkle in the olive oil, white wine vinegar, preserved lemons (if using), mint, and pistachios, and toss gently to mix. Season with salt and pepper. Set aside.

5. Heat a separate large skillet over medium-high heat until hot.

6. In a small bowl, combine the salt, cumin, coriander, ginger, and paprika.

7. Coat the salmon fillets with the remaining 2 tablespoons of coconut oil and season with the spice mixture, ½ teaspoon salt, and pepper.

8. Sear the salmon for about 2 minutes on each side, until it flakes easily with a fork but is still a deeper shade of pink on the inside. It will continue cooking once outside the pan.

9. Serve each salmon fillet alongside a serving of the cauliflower rice.

PER SERVING Calories: 409; Fat: 24g; Protein: 41g; Total Carbs: 10g; Fiber: 5g; Net Carbs: 5g
53% fat, 40% protein, 7% carbs

Spicy Italian Sausage and Mussels

KETO
QUOTIENT

 2 3

Serves 4 / Prep time: 10 minutes / Cook time: 18 to 20 minutes

NUT FREE • 30 MINUTES OR LESS

I enjoyed a dish similar to this one at a hilltop restaurant overlooking the San Pablo Bay, north of San Francisco. The spicy Italian sausage infused the broth and the mussels with an unforgettable flavor. Serve with Celery Root Purée (page 116).

2 tablespoons extra-virgin olive oil

8 ounces spicy Italian sausage, casings removed

1 medium onion, halved and thinly sliced

4 garlic cloves, smashed

½ cup dry red wine

2 tablespoons tomato paste

1 cup Chicken Bone Broth (page 224) or low-sodium chicken broth

2 pounds fresh mussels, scrubbed and de-bearded

Sea salt

Freshly ground black pepper

2 tablespoons cold butter, cut into pieces

1. Heat the olive oil in a large pot over medium heat.

2. Cook the sausage and onion for 7 to 8 minutes, until the sausage is gently browned and the onion begins to soften.

3. Add the garlic and cook for 30 seconds.

4. Add the wine and tomato paste and scrape the pan with a wooden spoon to remove the bits stuck to the bottom. Simmer for 2 minutes to burn off some of the alcohol.

5. Add the chicken broth and the mussels to the pot. Season with salt and pepper. Toss well, cover, and steam for 8 to 10 minutes, until all of the mussels have opened. Discard any that have not opened after 10 minutes. Remove cooked mussels, vegetables, and sausage to a serving dish.

6. Return the pot to the stove and simmer the cooking liquid until reduced to about 1 cup. Whisk in the butter 1 tablespoon at a time.

7. Pour the broth over the mussels, vegetables, and sausage.

PER SERVING Calories: 486; Fat: 29g; Protein: 36g; Total Carbs: 13g; Fiber: 1g; Net Carbs: 12g
59% fat, 30% protein, 11% carbs

Shrimp and Sausage Jambalaya

Serves 4 / Prep time: 10 minutes / Cook time: 18 to 20 minutes

DAIRY FREE • NUT FREE • 30 MINUTES OR LESS

Authentic Cajun jambalaya is made with white rice and is thickened with a roux, equal parts flour and butter (or oil) cooked until nutty and golden brown. This version skips the roux and the rice in favor of riced cauliflower. It may not be straight outta New Orleans, but it has a fraction of the carbs and calories of the original.

1 head cauliflower

¼ cup extra-virgin olive oil

½ cup diced yellow onion

½ cup diced green bell pepper

¼ cup diced celery stalk

1 teaspoon minced garlic

½ cup canned diced plum
   tomatoes, drained

1 pound andouille sausage

1 to 2 teaspoons Cajun seasoning

½ pound large shrimp, peeled
   and deveined

Sea salt

Freshly ground black pepper

2 tablespoons minced fresh parsley

1. In a food processor, pulse the cauliflower until coarsely ground, about the texture of rice.

2. Squeeze the cauliflower by the handful over the sink to remove excess moisture. Set aside.

3. In a large skillet, preferably cast iron, heat the olive oil over medium heat. Cook the onion, bell pepper, celery, and garlic until soft, about 10 minutes.

4. Add the tomatoes, and cook until most of the liquid has evaporated, about 2 minutes.

5. Add the sausage to the pan, and cook for 2 minutes.

6. Add the cauliflower and Cajun seasoning to the pan and sauté for 2 to 3 minutes.

7. Add the shrimp and continue cooking until the shrimp is cooked through, another 2 to 3 minutes.

8. Season with salt and pepper and garnish with parsley before serving.

PER SERVING Calories: 392; Fat: 26g; Protein: 30g; Total Carbs: 13g; Fiber: 5g; Net Carbs: 7g
60% fat, 31% protein, 9% carbs

INGREDIENT TIP: Make your own Cajun seasoning blend by combining 1 teaspoon each of garlic powder, onion powder, paprika, dried oregano, dried thyme, ground celery, cayenne, and black pepper. Use 1 teaspoon of the mixture in this recipe, and store the rest in a covered container.

Crab Cakes with Cilantro Crema

Serves 4 / Prep time: 10 minutes / Cook time: 15 to 18 minutes

30 MINUTES OR LESS

Traditional crab cakes are held together with lots of breadcrumbs, making them more bread cake than crab cake. This version uses egg and almond flour, which admittedly doesn't hold together as well when cooked in a pan. Baking in the oven makes them easier to handle.

¼ cup almond flour

1 egg, whisked

1 scallion, minced

1 garlic clove, minced

½ teaspoon sea salt

Pinch cayenne pepper

1 pound lump crabmeat,
   picked over for shells

1 tablespoon coconut oil

½ cup full-fat sour cream

½ cup full-fat mayonnaise

1 tablespoon lime juice

2 tablespoons minced cilantro

1. Preheat the oven to 375°F. Line a baking sheet with parchment paper.

2. In a medium bowl, whisk the almond flour, egg, scallion, garlic, sea salt, and cayenne pepper. Fold in the crabmeat.

3. Divide the mixture into 8 cakes and place them on the baking sheet. Brush with the oil. Bake for 15 to 18 minutes until the cakes are gently browned and set.

4. While the crab cakes bake, whisk together the sour cream, mayonnaise, lime juice, and cilantro in a jar to make the cilantro crema. Serve alongside the crab cakes.

PER SERVING Calories: 455; Fat: 36g; Protein: 30g; Total Carbs: 4g; Fiber: 1g; Net Carbs: 3g
71% fat, 26% protein, 3% carbs

VARIATION TIP: Make these cakes with canned cooked salmon and use fresh lemon juice and dill in the crema instead of lime and cilantro.

Vietnamese Shrimp Cakes

Serves 4 / Prep time: 10 minutes / Cook time: 5 minutes

DAIRY FREE • NUT FREE • 30 MINUTES OR LESS

Fragrant lemongrass, garlic, and red chile permeate these Vietnamese shrimp cakes. Traditionally, they're threaded onto sugarcane before being grilled or fried, and although that doesn't contribute many carbs to the recipe, they are tough to source even in Asian markets. To make this a complete meal, serve with the Sesame Ginger Slaw (page 93).

1 pound large shrimp, peeled
and deveined

1 tablespoon coconut flour

½ teaspoon sea salt

1 tablespoon minced lemongrass

1 teaspoon minced garlic

1 teaspoon minced red chile

¼ cup coconut oil

1. In a food processor, blend the shrimp, coconut flour, salt, lemongrass, garlic, and red chile until the mixture is thick but still slightly chunky.

2. Heat the coconut oil in a large skillet over medium-high heat until hot.

3. Form the shrimp mixture into small cakes, about 2 tablespoons each. Fry for 2 to 3 minutes on each side, until golden brown and cooked through.

PER SERVING Calories: 246; Fat: 16g; Protein: 23g; Total Carbs: 3g; Fiber: 1g; Net Carbs: 2g
59% fat, 37% protein, 4% carbs

INGREDIENT TIP: To prepare the lemongrass, remove the tough outer layers of the stalk and slice away the root end and nearly the whole tough end of the stalk. You should have a 2- to 3-inch segment. Slice into small rings to break up the fibers and then mince the rings. Alternatively, purchase a tube of puréed lemongrass from the produce section.

Sesame-Crusted Tuna
with Sweet Chili Vinaigrette

Serves 4 / Prep time: 10 minutes / Cook time: 5 minutes

DAIRY FREE • NUT FREE • 30 MINUTES OR LESS

Most sweet chili sauce recipes are thickened with cornstarch and sweetened with sugar, making them unsuitable for keto diets. This version functions more like a vinaigrette, combining the traditional flavors of Thai chili sauce and rice wine vinegar, lightly sweetened with stevia.

1 tablespoon Thai chili sauce, such as sambal

1 tablespoon rice wine vinegar

¼ cup light olive oil or canola oil

4 to 6 drops liquid stevia

4 (6-ounce) ahi tuna steaks

2 tablespoons toasted sesame oil

Sea salt

Freshly ground black pepper

½ cup sesame seeds

4 packed cups mixed spring greens

1. In a jar, combine the chili sauce, vinegar, oil, and stevia. Cover tightly with a lid and shake vigorously. Set aside.

2. Preheat a large skillet over medium-high heat.

3. Pat the tuna steaks dry with paper towels. Coat each side of the steaks with the sesame oil, and season with the salt and pepper.

4. Spread the sesame seeds in a shallow dish. Press the tuna steaks into the seeds to coat them on both sides.

5. Immediately place the tuna steaks into the hot skillet. Sear on each side for 1½ minutes for rare.

6. Divide the greens among the serving plates and drizzle each salad with the chili vinaigrette.

7. Transfer the tuna to a cutting board and slice each steak on an angle into ½-inch pieces. It will still be dark and barely warm in the center. Place equal portions of the tuna on each serving plate.

PER SERVING Calories: 475; Fat: 32g; Protein: 41g; Total Carbs: 11g; Fiber: 3g; Net Carbs: 8g
60% fat, 32% protein, 8% carbs

INGREDIENT TIP: Tuna is best served rare or medium-rare, so purchase sushi-grade tuna. You can find this available at good-quality fish markets or in the frozen section of well-stocked grocery stores. When buying frozen, choose vacuum-sealed ahi tuna for the best quality. Defrost in cold water for 1 hour or until thawed before preparing this recipe.

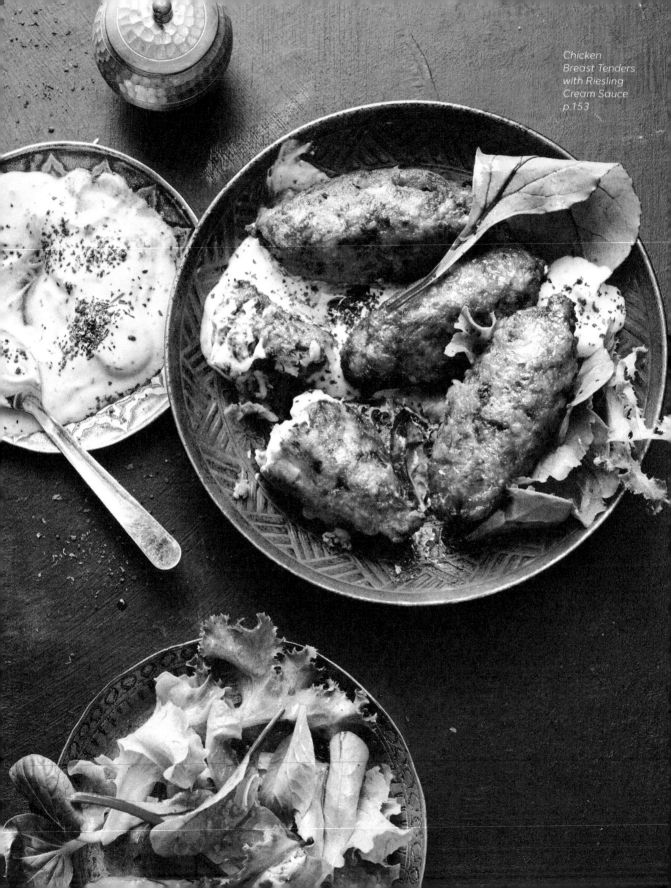

Chicken
Breast Tenders
with Riesling
Cream Sauce
p.153

CHAPTER NINE
Chicken

Essential Roasted Chicken

Serves 4 / Prep time: 5 minutes / Cook time: 30 to 35 minutes

DAIRY FREE • NUT FREE

Using the whole bird saves money, and you can make a killer Chicken Bone Broth (page 224) with the leftover carcass. To make this a complete meal, add a few vegetables such as onions, zucchini, and carrots to the pan. For an even roasting time and maximum crispy skin, I remove the backbone from the chicken and cook it "spatchcock" style, as described in this recipe.

1 whole chicken, about 3 to 4 pounds

1 garlic clove, halved

2 tablespoons coconut oil or
   bacon grease

Sea salt

Freshly ground black pepper

1. Preheat the oven to 375°F.

2. Stand the chicken on one end and use a serrated knife to cut down one side of the backbone and then the other. Spread the chicken open on the roasting pan and flatten the breasts with the palm of your hand.

3. Pat the chicken dry with paper towels and then rub with the cut garlic clove on all sides. Coat the chicken with the oil or grease, and then season generously with salt and pepper, making sure to season the underside of the bird as well.

4. Roast for 30 to 35 minutes, basting once or twice with the rendered fat and pan juices, until the chicken is cooked through to an internal temperature of 165°F.

PER SERVING Calories: 490; Fat: 30g; Protein: 51g; Total Carbs: 0g; Fiber: 0g; Net Carbs: 0g
55% fat, 45% protein, 0% carbs

VARIATION TIP: Coat the chicken with 2 tablespoons of minced herbs, such as thyme and rosemary, before roasting.

Roasted Chicken and Zucchini with Wine Reduction

Serves 4 / Prep time: 10 minutes / Cook time: 30 to 32 minutes

NUT FREE

Sometimes the tastiest recipes are also the simplest. This hearty main dish involves multiple cooking techniques designed to transform every-day ingredients into something spectacular. Serve alone or with Celery Root Purée (page 116) or Mashed Cauliflower (page 219) for an unforgettable meal.

2 tablespoons coconut oil

8 bone-in, skin-on chicken thighs

Sea salt

Freshly ground black pepper

2 medium zucchini, halved lengthwise and cut into 1-inch pieces

1 teaspoon minced fresh thyme

½ cup dry red wine

3 tablespoons cold butter, cut into pieces

1. Preheat the oven to 400°F.

2. Heat a large ovenproof skillet over medium-high heat. Melt the coconut oil in the skillet.

3. Pat the chicken thighs dry with paper towels. Season generously with salt and pepper.

4. Place the chicken thighs skin-side down in the skillet, and cook for 5 to 7 minutes, until a crispy skin develops.

5. Flip the chicken, and add the zucchini and thyme to the skillet. Transfer the skillet to the oven and bake for 20 minutes, or until the chicken is cooked through to an internal temperature of 165°F.

6. Transfer the chicken and zucchini to individual serving plates. Using potholders, return the skillet to the stove top, taking care with the very hot pan.

continued >

7. Pour the red wine into the skillet and simmer over medium heat until reduced by half, about 5 minutes. Remove the skillet from the heat.

8. Whisk in the cold butter 1 tablespoon at a time. The sauce will become thick and glossy.

9. Drizzle the sauce around the chicken and zucchini.

PER SERVING Calories: 490; Fat: 34g; Protein: 36g; Total Carbs: 5g; Fiber: 1g; Net Carbs: 4g
64% fat, 32% protein, 4% carbs

Chicken Breast Tenders
with Riesling Cream Sauce

Serves 4 / Prep time: 10 minutes / Cook time: 28 to 30 minutes

NUT FREE

It doesn't get much more indulgent than chicken breast coated in a thick Riesling cream sauce. This chicken dish is delicious served with Caramelized Fennel (page 122) and Stuffed Mushrooms (page 119).

4 (about 6-ounce) boneless, skinless
   chicken breasts

½ cup almond flour

2 tablespoons coconut flour

1 teaspoon garlic powder

Sea salt

Freshly ground pepper

2 tablespoons canola oil

½ cup Riesling or Sauvignon Blanc

½ cup Chicken Bone Broth (page 224)

½ cup heavy cream

4 cups mixed greens

1. Preheat the oven to 250°F.

2. Slice the chicken into 4-by-2-inch pieces.

3. In a shallow dish, mix together the almond flour, coconut flour, garlic powder, salt, and pepper. Dredge the chicken pieces in the flour mixture.

4. Heat the canola oil in a large skillet over medium-high heat. Sear the chicken pieces for 2 to 3 minutes on each side until well browned. Transfer to a baking dish and place in the oven to keep warm.

5. Add the Riesling to the pan and cook until reduced to about ¼ cup, about 3 minutes. Add the broth and heavy cream, and cook over medium-low heat to thicken the sauce for 5 minutes.

6. Place the chicken onto serving plates and garnish with the mixed greens. Serve the Riesling cream sauce on the side.

PER SERVING Calories: 475; Fat: 30g; Protein: 43g; Total Carbs: 7g; Fiber: 4g; Net Carbs: 3g
57% fat, 36% protein, 7% carbs

Curried Chicken Salad

Serves 4 / Prep time: 10 minutes / Cook time: 0 minutes

DAIRY FREE • 30 MINUTES OR LESS

Use leftovers from the Essential Roasted Chicken (page 150) here. Alternatively, purchase a rotisserie chicken from the deli section of the supermarket. This curried chicken salad can be served on its own or used to fill lettuce cups.

½ cup full-fat mayonnaise

1 tablespoon lemon juice

1 teaspoon curry powder

Sea salt

Freshly ground black pepper

16 ounces shredded cooked chicken, light and dark meat

¼ cup roughly chopped toasted cashews

1 celery stalk, minced

¼ cup diced red onion

1. In a medium mixing bowl, whisk together the mayonnaise, lemon juice, and curry powder. Season with salt and pepper.

2. Fold in the chicken, cashews, celery, and red onion. Serve immediately or refrigerate until ready to serve.

PER SERVING Calories: 379; Fat: 28g; Protein: 27g; Total Carbs: 4g; Fiber: 1g; Net Carbs: 3g
67% fat, 29% protein, 4% carbs

Crispy Chicken Paillard

Serves 4 / Prep time: 10 minutes / Cook time: 10 minutes

30 MINUTES OR LESS

KETO
QUOTIENT

① 2 3

The literal French translation of paillard *has connotations of locker room bawdiness, so I have no idea how it came to mean a cut of meat pounded to a uniform thinness before cooking. Whatever its etymology, the method yields a delicious, perfectly cooked chicken breast and solves the problem of the meat being overcooked on the outside and undercooked in the center.*

½ cup grated Parmesan cheese

¼ cup almond flour

1 teaspoon garlic powder

½ teaspoon sea salt

½ teaspoon freshly ground
   black pepper

4 boneless 6-ounce chicken breasts

2 tablespoons canola oil

1. Mix the Parmesan cheese, almond flour, garlic powder, salt, and pepper in a shallow dish.

2. Place the chicken breasts one at a time between two sheets of parchment paper. Pound with the flat side of a meat mallet until the chicken is about ¼-inch thick all the way through, being careful not to pound right through the chicken.

3. Heat the canola oil in a large skillet over medium-high heat.

4. Lightly coat the chicken pieces in the Parmesan and flour mixture, and sear for 5 minutes on each side, or until just cooked through.

PER SERVING Calories: 362; Fat: 19g; Protein: 45g; Total Carbs: 2g; Fiber: 1g; Net Carbs: 1g
48% fat, 50% protein, 2% carbs

Tomato Basil Chicken Zoodle Bowls

Serves 4 / Prep time: 20 minutes / Cook time: 7 to 10 minutes

NUT FREE • 30 MINUTES OR LESS

This dish is perfect for late summer when you want something light and flavorful that makes good use of what's in season. The first time I had this dish, it was completely vegetarian, so omit the chicken and double the mozzarella if you want to go meatless for a meal.

2 medium zucchini

Sea salt

Freshly ground black pepper

4 tablespoons extra-virgin
   olive oil, divided

1 pound chicken thighs, cut into
   1-inch pieces

½ cup roughly chopped fresh basil

1 pint grape tomatoes, halved

1 garlic clove, minced

8 ounces fresh mozzarella,
   cut into ½-inch pieces

1. Cut off the stem ends of the zucchini. Place the cut sides on the spiralizer blade and firmly attach the spiky end of the spiralizer to the opposite end of the zucchini. Run the zucchini through the spiralizer to produce long, thin noodles.

2. Place the zucchini noodles into a colander and season very generously with salt. Place the colander into the sink and let the zucchini sweat for 20 minutes.

3. Rinse the zucchini with fresh water and wring as much moisture as you can from the noodles, trying not to break them.

4. Heat a large skillet over high heat. Season the chicken generously with salt and pepper. When the pan is hot, add 2 tablespoons of the olive oil. When the oil is hot, cook the chicken for 5 to 7 minutes, or until gently browned and cooked through. Transfer to a large serving dish.

5. In the same pan, sauté the zucchini noodles for 2 to 3 minutes, or until hot but not browned.

6. Transfer the cooked zucchini to the serving dish along with the basil, tomatoes, garlic, and fresh mozzarella. Give everything a good toss, drizzle with the remaining olive oil, and season with salt and pepper.

PER SERVING Calories: 456; Fat: 31g; Protein: 37g; Total Carbs: 6g; Fiber: 1g; Net Carbs: 5g
61% fat, 32% protein, 7% carbs

Carne Asada Chicken Bowls

Serves 4 / Prep time: 10 minutes / Cook time: 25 minutes

DAIRY FREE • NUT FREE

I love the contrasts of flavors and textures in this simple dish. Instead of carb-loaded rice, which is a traditional backdrop for lunch bowls, this recipe uses cauliflower rice. You could also opt for shredded cabbage, lettuce, and cilantro. If you have the time, marinate the chicken for up to 8 hours in the refrigerator before baking.

4 tablespoons extra-virgin
   olive oil, divided

2 tablespoons low-sodium soy sauce

2 tablespoons lime juice

½ cup minced fresh cilantro

2 garlic cloves, minced

1 teaspoon ground cumin

1 teaspoon smoked paprika

¼ teaspoon cayenne pepper

16 ounces boneless, skinless
   chicken thighs

1 small head of cauliflower,
   broken into florets

1 tablespoon coconut oil

1 avocado, pitted, peeled, and sliced

½ cup sour cream

4 radishes, thinly sliced

1. Preheat the oven to 350°F.

2. In a small baking dish, mix together 3 tablespoons of the olive oil, soy sauce, lime juice, cilantro, garlic, cumin, paprika, and cayenne. Add the chicken to the dish and coat thoroughly in the mixture. Bake for 25 minutes, or until the chicken is cooked through. Use a fork to shred the chicken.

3. While the chicken bakes, pulse the cauliflower in a food processor until coarsely ground, about the texture of rice.

4. Squeeze the cauliflower by the handful over the sink to remove excess moisture.

5. Heat the remaining tablespoon of oil in a large skillet over medium-high heat, and stir-fry the cauliflower for 5 minutes, until just heated through.

6. Divide the cauliflower rice among the serving dishes. Place equal portions of the cooked chicken along with some of the pan juices over the rice. Top each serving with a quarter of the avocado slices, sour cream, and radish slices.

PER SERVING Calories: 422; Fat: 31g; Protein: 28g; Total Carbs: 9g; Fiber: 5g; Net Carbs: 4g
66% fat, 27% protein, 7% carbs

Spaghetti Squash Chicken Bowls

Serves 4 / Prep time: 10 minutes / Cook time: 30 minutes

DAIRY FREE

As its name suggests, spaghetti squash is a vegetable that has the texture of pasta. You don't need any special equipment, either. Simply slice, roast, and marvel at this squash's noodle-like texture. This dish is also good with a handful of steamed broccoli florets for color.

1 small spaghetti squash

2 tablespoons canola oil, divided

1½ pounds boneless, skinless chicken
  thighs, cut into 2-inch pieces

Sea salt

Freshly ground black pepper

1 teaspoon minced ginger

1 teaspoon minced garlic

Pinch red pepper flakes

2 tablespoons toasted sesame oil

¼ cup low-sodium soy sauce

Juice of 1 lime

¼ cup roasted cashews

1. Preheat the oven to 375°F.

2. Slice the spaghetti squash into 1-inch-thick rings, and scoop out the strings and seeds. Place the squash rings onto a rimmed baking sheet and brush with 1 tablespoon of the canola oil. Roast for 30 minutes, until the squash is tender.

3. While the squash is roasting, heat the remaining tablespoon of oil in a large skillet. Season the chicken with salt and pepper. Sear the chicken in the pan, and cook for 5 to 7 minutes, or until it is well browned and cooked through.

4. Add the ginger, garlic, and red pepper flakes to the pan and cook for 30 seconds. Remove the pan from the heat.

5. When the spaghetti squash rings are cool enough to handle, use a fork to shred the flesh into long, thin strands. Divide the squash among the serving bowls, and top with equal portions of the cooked chicken.

6. In a small measuring cup, whisk together the sesame oil, soy sauce, and lime juice. Pour the sauce over the spaghetti squash bowls and top with the roasted cashews.

PER SERVING Calories: 440; Fat: 25g; Protein: 40g; Total Carbs: 13g; Fiber: 2g; Net Carbs: 11g
51% fat, 36% protein, 13% carbs

INGREDIENT TIP: Slicing the spaghetti squash crosswise in rings yields longer strands of "spaghetti" than slicing the squash in half lengthwise.

Thai Chicken Lettuce Cups

Serves 4 / Prep time: 10 minutes / Cook time: 10 minutes

DAIRY FREE • 30 MINUTES OR LESS

These flavorful lettuce cups with spicy peanut sauce are so delicious, I could almost eat the whole batch by myself! For a filling takeout-style menu, serve these lettuce cups with Cauliflower Rice (page 218) topped with lime zest.

2 tablespoons toasted sesame oil

2 tablespoons canola oil

1 pound boneless, skinless chicken thighs, finely diced

8 ounces button mushrooms, finely diced

2 teaspoons minced ginger, divided

2 teaspoons minced garlic, divided

Sea salt

Freshly ground black pepper

3 tablespoons low-sodium soy sauce, divided

Juice of 1 lime

⅓ cup natural peanut butter

Pinch red pepper flakes

8 to 12 butter lettuce leaves

¼ cup roughly chopped roasted peanuts

¼ cup grated carrot

1 scallion, thinly sliced

1. Heat the sesame oil and canola oil in a large skillet over medium-high heat. Add the chicken and mushrooms, and sauté until cooked through and well-browned, about 10 minutes.

2. Add 1 teaspoon each of the ginger and garlic and cook for another 30 seconds. Stir in 1 tablespoon of soy sauce. Remove the pan from the heat. Season with salt and pepper.

3. Meanwhile, combine the remaining 1 teaspoon of ginger, remaining 1 teaspoon of garlic, remaining 2 tablespoons of soy sauce, peanut butter, lime juice, and red pepper flakes in a small jar. Cover tightly with a lid and shake vigorously. Thin with 2 to 3 tablespoons of water until it reaches the desired consistency.

4. To serve, place a spoonful of the chicken mushroom mixture into each lettuce cup. Top with a pinch of peanuts, carrot, and scallion. Serve with the peanut sauce.

PER SERVING Calories: 490; Fat: 34g; Protein: 35g; Total Carbs: 12g; Fiber: 3g; Net Carbs: 9g 62% fat, 29% protein, 9% carbs

VARIATION TIP: For a vegan version of these lettuce cups, use 16 ounces of pressed, crumbled tofu in place of the chicken.

VARIATION PER SERVING Calories: 428; Fat: 34g; Protein: 21g; Total Carbs: 14g; Fiber: 1g; Net Carbs: 13g; 71% fat, 20% protein, 13% carbs

Chicken Cordon Bleu

Serves 4 / Prep time: 5 minutes / Cook time: 25 minutes

30 MINUTES OR LESS

In French, cordon bleu *means "blue ribbon," indicating the highest quality, so it feels a little like cheating to turn this classic stuffed chicken dish into a casserole. But sometimes the best meals are those that require the least amount of effort. The almond flour and Parmesan cheese form a deliciously crispy topping for the melted cheese, prosciutto, and chicken.*

1 tablespoon butter

1 pound boneless, skinless
   chicken thighs

2 teaspoons Dijon mustard

Sea salt

Freshly ground black pepper

4 ounces prosciutto or deli ham,
   roughly chopped

4 ounces sliced Swiss cheese

½ cup almond flour

½ cup grated Parmesan cheese

1. Preheat the oven to 400°F. Coat the interior of an 8-by-8-inch baking dish with butter.

2. Coat the chicken thighs with the mustard, and season with salt and pepper. Place the chicken into the baking dish.

3. Top the chicken with the prosciutto. Spread the Swiss cheese slices over the prosciutto layer.

4. In a bowl, mix together the almond flour, Parmesan cheese, and paprika. Sprinkle this mixture over the cheese and season with salt and pepper.

5. Bake for 25 minutes or until the chicken is cooked through and the top is browned and bubbling.

PER SERVING Calories: 476; Fat: 31g; Protein: 45g; Total Carbs: 5g; Fiber: 2g; Net Carbs: 3g
59% fat, 37% protein, 4% carbs

PREP TIP: This recipe is easily doubled to feed a crowd or divided into individual baking dishes for easy meal prep.

Chicken with Mushrooms, Port, and Cream

Serves 4 / Prep time: 10 minutes / Cook time: 20 minutes

NUT FREE • 30 MINUTES OR LESS

The so-called French paradox refers to the thinness of French people despite a menu laden with heavy cream and butter. So it's only fitting that this book includes some classic French recipes. I've simplified this one to make an easy weeknight supper you can prepare in fewer than 30 minutes from grocery bag to dinner table. Serve with Celery Root Purée (page 116) and steamed vegetables for a complete meal.

2 tablespoons canola oil	1 shallot, minced
8 boneless, skinless chicken thighs	8 ounces mushrooms, sliced
Sea salt	¼ cup port wine
Freshly ground black pepper	½ cup heavy cream

1. Heat the canola oil in a large skillet over medium-high heat. Pat the chicken thighs dry with paper towels and season generously with salt and pepper.

2. Sear the chicken thighs on each side until well browned and cooked through to an internal temperature of 165°F, about 8 minutes. Transfer them to a separate dish. Add the shallot and mushrooms to the pan and cook for 10 minutes, until the mushrooms are browned and most of the moisture has evaporated from the pan.

3. Add the port and cook until reduced to just a couple of tablespoons, about 2 minutes.

continued >

Chicken with Mushrooms, Port, and Cream *continued*

4. Stir in the heavy cream and bring to the barest simmer. Return the chicken thighs to the pan, basting with the cream sauce. Season with salt and pepper.

PER SERVING Calories: 389; Fat: 24g; Protein: 30g; Total Carbs: 6g; Fiber: 1g; Net Carbs: 5g
61% fat, 33% protein, 6% carbs

SUBSTITUTION TIP: If you want to skip the port wine, go for it. You can omit it entirely or use dry sherry, white or red wine, or even a tablespoon of wine vinegar to deglaze the pan. Just make sure to reduce it for a few minutes before stirring in the cream.

Chicken Adobo

Serves 4 / Prep time: 5 minutes / Cook time: 33 to 36 minutes

KETO
QUOTIENT

① 2 3

DAIRY FREE • NUT FREE

This Filipino dish is loaded with flavor from smashed garlic, black pepper, soy sauce, and rice vinegar. Traditionally the peppercorns are left whole, so feel free to do that if you like. I find it easier to eat if I'm not dodging little fireballs. Serve it with Cauliflower Rice (page 218) or with a simple side salad.

2 tablespoons canola oil

4 bone-in, skin-on chicken leg
   and thighs

Sea salt

Freshly ground black pepper

6 garlic cloves, smashed

½ cup rice vinegar

⅓ cup low-sodium soy sauce

½ cup Chicken Bone Broth (page 224)
   or low-sodium chicken broth

2 bay leaves

1 scallion, thinly sliced

1. Preheat the oven to 400°F.

2. Heat a large cast iron or other ovenproof skillet over medium-high heat. Heat the oil until it shimmers.

3. Pat the chicken pieces dry with paper towels and season generously with salt and pepper.

4. Place the chicken skin-side down into the pan and sear for 7 to 10 minutes, until it gets a nice, brown crust. Flip the chicken.

5. Add the garlic to the pan, and cook for 1 minute. Stir in the rice vinegar, soy sauce, chicken broth, and bay leaves, and bring to a simmer.

6. Transfer the pan to the oven and cook for another 25 minutes until the chicken is cooked through to an internal temperature of 165°F. Garnish with scallions just before serving.

PER SERVING Calories: 392; Fat: 25g; Protein: 36g; Total Carbs: 3g; Fiber: 0g; Net Carbs: 3g
58% fat, 37% protein, 5% carbs

Chorizo, Chicken, and Salsa Verde

Serves 4 / Prep time: 20 minutes / Cook time: 40 to 43 minutes

DAIRY FREE • NUT FREE

The first time I made this dish, I was undone with how good it tasted. The savory chicken and spicy chorizo perfectly balance with the cool, tangy salsa verde. It has more calories than some of the other recipes in this chapter, but it is low in carbs.

2 tablespoons canola oil

1 pound bone-in, skin-on
   chicken thighs

1 tablespoon good-quality
   chili powder

Sea salt

Freshly ground black pepper

8 ounces chorizo

1 onion, roughly chopped

1 cup canned plum tomatoes,
   hand crushed

2 cups Chicken Bone Broth (page 224)

1 jalapeño pepper

1 cup minced fresh cilantro

¼ cup extra-virgin olive oil

2 tablespoons lime juice

¼ teaspoon sea salt

1 bay leaf

1. Preheat the oven to 400°F.

2. Heat a large cast iron or other ovenproof skillet over medium-high heat. Heat the canola oil.

3. Pat the chicken pieces dry with paper towels and season with the chili powder, salt, and pepper.

4. Place the chicken skin-side down in the skillet and sear for 7 to 10 minutes, until it gets a nice, brown crust. Flip the chicken and sear for about 3 minutes on the bottom side. Transfer the partially cooked chicken to a separate dish.

5. Add the chorizo to the skillet and cook until just browned. Transfer it to the dish with the chicken.

6. Add the onion and garlic to the skillet and cook for 10 minutes, until soft. Add the plum tomatoes, chicken broth, and bay leaf. Bring to a simmer.

7. Return the chicken pieces and chorizo to the skillet and transfer to the oven. Bake for 20 minutes, or until the chicken is cooked through to an internal temperature of 165°F and the stewed tomatoes and onions are thick and rich. Remove and discard the bay leaf.

8. While the chicken is baking, combine the cilantro, jalapeño, olive oil, lime juice, and salt in a blender. Purée until the mixture is mostly smooth.

9. To serve, scoop a quarter of the tomato and onion mixture into four serving bowls. Top with a piece of chicken and drizzle with the salsa verde.

PER SERVING Calories: 661; Fat: 52g; Protein: 40g; Total Carbs: 8g; Fiber: 2g; Net Carbs: 6g
71% fat, 24% protein, 5% carbs

INGREDIENT TIP: Make your own chili powder by combining 1 tablespoon each of ground ancho chili, ground cumin, and smoked paprika with 1 teaspoon each of garlic powder, onion powder, and dried oregano.

Tandoori Vegetable Chicken Skewers

Serves 4 / Prep time: 10 minutes, plus 15 minutes marinating time
Cook time: 15 minutes

NUT FREE

Turmeric gives tandoori chicken its brilliant yellow hue, but if you like it hot (and bright red), increase the cayenne pepper. It is served with a simple side salad of arugula, red onions, and grape tomatoes. It is also lovely with Cauliflower Rice (page 218).

½ cup full-fat yogurt

2 tablespoons lemon juice

1 tablespoon minced garlic

1 teaspoon ground turmeric

1 teaspoon ground coriander

1 teaspoon ground cumin

1 teaspoon garam masala

¼ teaspoon cayenne pepper

1½ pounds boneless, skinless chicken thighs, cut into 2-inch pieces

2 tablespoons canola oil

1 green bell pepper, seeds and ribs removed, cut into 2-inch pieces

1 yellow bell pepper, seeds and ribs removed, cut into 2-inch pieces

1 red onion

Sea salt

Freshly ground black pepper

2 tablespoons white wine vinegar

¼ cup extra virgin olive oil

4 cups arugula

1 cup grape tomatoes, halved

1 tablespoon sesame seeds

1. Preheat an outdoor grill or a grill pan to medium-high.

2. In a large glass bowl, whisk together the yogurt, lemon juice, garlic, turmeric, coriander, cumin, garam masala, and cayenne pepper.

3. Add the chicken thighs to the yogurt mixture and toss to coat. Allow the chicken to marinate for at least 15 minutes.

4. Slice the onion in half and then slice each half into four pieces, reserving two for the salad.

5. Thread the chicken, green and yellow peppers, and red onion onto bamboo or wooden skewers. Brush the vegetables with the canola oil (some will get onto the chicken, and that's okay). Season generously with salt and pepper.

6. Grill the skewers for about 15 minutes total, turning the skewers as you go so the chicken and vegetables are gently browned on all sides.

7. Meanwhile, whisk the white wine vinegar and olive oil in a large mixing bowl. Slice the remaining red onion into thin pieces and toss with the arugula and tomatoes in the vinaigrette.

8. Divide the salad and grilled chicken skewers among the serving plates, and sprinkle each with an equal portion of the sesame seeds.

PER SERVING Calories: 463; Fat: 30g; Protein: 39g; Total Carbs: 8g; Fiber: 1g; Net Carbs: 7g
58% fat, 37% protein, 5% carbs

INGREDIENT TIP: If you have time, allow the chicken to marinate in the mixture for up to 8 hours for even more flavor.

Kung Pao Chicken

Serves 4 / Prep time: 5 minutes / Cook time: 15 minutes

DAIRY FREE • 30 MINUTES OR LESS

"Numbing" is a common description given to authentic Kung Pao chicken, and it comes from the judicious use of Sichuan peppercorns, which are available in Asian markets, online, or in well-stocked grocery stores. Serve this chicken dish with Cauliflower Rice (page 218). If you are sensitive to gluten, use balsamic vinegar instead of the Chinese black vinegar, which contains barley malt.

½ teaspoon ground Sichuan peppercorns

2 tablespoons low-sodium soy sauce

2 tablespoons Chinese black vinegar or balsamic vinegar

1 tablespoon rice wine or dry sherry

1 teaspoon toasted sesame oil

3 tablespoons canola oil

1½ pounds boneless, skinless chicken thighs, cut into 2-inch pieces

Sea salt

Freshly ground black pepper

1 red bell pepper, seeds and ribs removed, cut into 1-inch pieces

4 scallions, white and pale green parts only, thinly sliced

1 teaspoon minced garlic

1 teaspoon minced ginger

¼ teaspoon red pepper flakes

½ cup peanuts

1. In a jar, combine the Sichuan pepper, soy sauce, vinegar, rice wine or sherry, and sesame oil. Cover tightly with a lid and shake vigorously. Set aside.

2. Heat the canola oil in a large skillet over medium-high heat. Season the chicken generously with salt and pepper. Sauté the chicken in the hot oil until just cooked through to an internal temperature of 165°F, about 10 minutes. Transfer the chicken to a separate dish.

3. Cook the bell pepper and scallions in the same skillet for 3 minutes, or until crisp-tender. Add the scallions, garlic, ginger, and red pepper flakes to the skillet and cook for 30 seconds, just until fragrant.

4. Return the cooked chicken and any accumulated juices to the pan and add the Sichuan pepper sauce. Cook for 1 minute to allow the flavors to come together. Garnish each portion with a quarter of the peanuts.

PER SERVING Calories: 451; Fat: 27g; Protein: 42g; Total Carbs: 10g; Fiber: 3g; Net Carbs: 7g
54% fat, 37% protein, 9% carbs

SUBSTITUTION TIP: Sichuan peppercorns are also called Chinese coriander. Although not identical in flavor, a blend of regular black peppercorns and coriander can stand in.

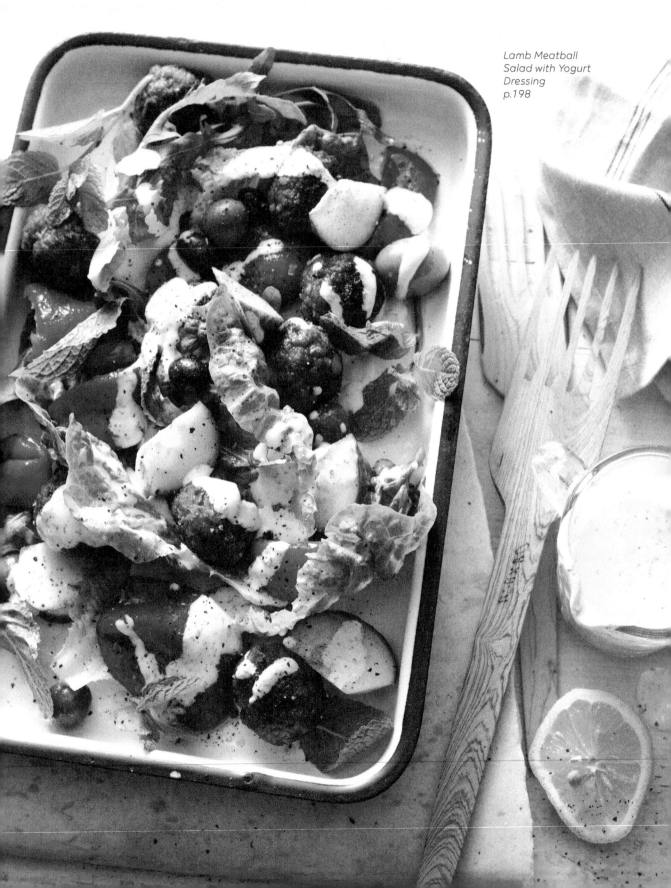

Lamb Meatball
Salad with Yogurt
Dressing
p.198

CHAPTER TEN
Beef, Lamb & Pork

Loaded Burgers

KETO
QUOTIENT

1 ② 3

Serves 4 / Prep time: 5 minutes / Cook time: 20 minutes

DAIRY FREE • NUT FREE • 30 MINUTES OR LESS

Bun-less cheeseburgers are a low-carb diet staple, but they can easily become boring. I spiced things up by adding caramelized onions, tomatoes, and a tangy chipotle mayonnaise. After enjoying burgers wrapped in lettuce for so long, I've come to actually prefer them this way—the sauce doesn't get soaked up in the bun, so you really get to enjoy it.

1 tablespoon canola oil

1 yellow onion, halved and thinly sliced

Pinch salt

¼ cup full-fat mayonnaise

2 tablespoons ketchup

1 teaspoon adobo sauce from
   canned chipotles

1 pound ground beef

Sea salt

Freshly ground black pepper

1 head iceberg or butter lettuce

1 beefsteak tomato, cut into
   4 thick slices

1. Heat the canola oil in a large skillet over medium heat. Cook the onion with a pinch of salt until soft and browned, about 20 minutes.

2. While the onion cooks, whisk together the mayonnaise, ketchup, and adobo sauce in a small measuring cup.

3. Preheat an outdoor grill or a grill pan to medium heat. Shape the ground beef into 4 patties. Season generously with salt and pepper. Grill for 4 minutes on each side for medium-rare, or longer depending on your desired level of doneness.

4. Break apart the lettuce into 8 large leaves. Top each leaf with a burger patty, followed by a spoonful of the chipotle mayonnaise, a slice of tomato, and the caramelized onions. Top with the remaining lettuce leaf.

PER SERVING Calories: 425; Fat: 35g; Protein: 21g; Total Carbs: 8g; Fiber: 1g; Net Carbs: 7g
74% fat, 20% protein, 6% carbs

VARIATION TIP: Some other delicious low-carb burger fixin's include cooked bacon, sliced cheese, seared mushrooms, and avocado. Keep in mind that additional toppings will change the nutrient profile.

Beef and Broccoli

Serves 4 / Prep time: 10 minutes / Cook time: 12 minutes

DAIRY FREE • NUT FREE • 30 MINUTES OR LESS

This Chinese takeout standby gets a healthy, low-carb makeover, forgoing the cornstarch and sugar found in many restaurant options. Serve it with Cauliflower Rice (page 218) for a complete meal.

2 tablespoons toasted sesame oil

3 tablespoons canola oil

1 pound boneless sirloin, cut in
   paper-thin slices

Sea salt

Freshly ground black pepper

2 tablespoons minced ginger

2 teaspoons minced garlic

Pinch red pepper flakes

1 head broccoli, cut into florets
   and stalks, diced

¼ cup low-sodium soy sauce

2 tablespoons dry sherry

1. Heat the sesame oil and canola oil in a large wok or skillet over medium-high heat until very hot.

2. Season the sirloin generously with salt and pepper.

3. Stir-fry the sirloin until just cooked through, about 5 minutes. Add the ginger, garlic, and red pepper flakes and cook for 1 minute, just until fragrant. Transfer the beef to a separate dish with a slotted spoon.

4. Add the broccoli to the pan and stir-fry for 5 minutes, until bright green and crisp tender.

5. Return the beef and any accumulated juices to the pan, and add the soy sauce and sherry. Simmer for 2 minutes until the liquid has reduced and the beef and broccoli are coated in the sauce.

PER SERVING Calories: 472; Fat: 29g; Protein: 41g; Total Carbs: 12g; Fiber: 5g; Net Carbs: 7g
55% fat, 35% protein, 10% carbs

INGREDIENT TIP: Freeze the beef for 20 minutes before slicing to get the thinnest slices possible.

Essential New York Strip Steak

Serves 4 / Prep time: 5 minutes / Cook time: 10 to 12 minutes

NUT FREE • 30 MINUTES OR LESS

*This is one of the easiest recipes in this book, but when cooked well
(not to be confused with well-done), it's one of the tastiest. Serve it with
Pan-Roasted Brussels Sprouts with Bacon (page 112) and Celery Root
Purée (page 116) for a decadent low-carb dinner.*

1 tablespoon coconut oil

4 (6-ounce) New York strip steaks

Sea salt

Freshly ground black pepper

¼ cup butter, at room temperature

1 tablespoon minced shallots

1 tablespoon minced rosemary

1. Preheat the oven to 350°F. Heat a large skillet over medium-high heat.
    Add the coconut oil.

2. Pat the steaks dry with paper towels and season generously with salt
    and pepper. Sear the steaks for about 5 minutes, then flip and sear for
    another 2 minutes before transferring the skillet to the oven. Continue
    cooking in the oven for about 3 minutes for medium-rare or 5 minutes
    for medium.

3. While the steak is cooking, make a simple compound butter by mashing
    together the butter, shallots, and rosemary.

4. To serve, top each steak with a tablespoon of the compound butter.

PER SERVING Calories: 473; Fat: 36g; Protein: 38g; Total Carbs: 1g; Fiber: 0g; Net Carbs: 1g
68% fat, 32% protein, <1% carbs

INGREDIENT TIP: Double the compound butter recipe and store it in the refrigerator to add to all kinds of dishes to increase flavor and up the fat ratio.

Meatloaf

KETO
QUOTIENT

1 ② 3

Serves 8 / Prep time: 15 minutes / Cook time: 1 hour

DAIRY FREE

Meatloaf is such a comforting dish, and this version uses almond flour and diced tomatoes instead of breadcrumbs. Unlike bunless hamburgers, where you know something's missing, meatloaf is perfectly complete with nothing more than a handful of green beans and a glass of red wine. Then again, it also goes well with a generous dollop of Mashed Cauliflower (page 219).

1 tablespoon canola oil

1 cup minced onion

1 teaspoon minced garlic

1 teaspoon minced rosemary

¼ cup roughly chopped parsley

½ cup diced tomatoes,
   fresh or canned

½ cup almond flour

2 tablespoons tomato paste

1 egg, whisked

1 teaspoon sea salt

1 teaspoon freshly ground
   black pepper

1 pound ground beef

1 pound ground pork

4 slices raw bacon

1. Preheat the oven to 350°F.

2. Heat the canola oil in a skillet over medium heat. Cook the onion, garlic, rosemary, and parsley for 8 to 10 minutes, until soft. Stir in the tomatoes. Remove the pan from the heat.

3. In a large mixing bowl, whisk together the almond flour, tomato paste, egg, salt, and pepper until a thick paste is formed.

4. Add the beef and pork to the cooked onions. Using your hands, mix the ingredients until just combined; do not overmix.

5. Transfer the meat mixture to a loaf pan, and top with the bacon slices. Bake for 1 hour or until the meatloaf is cooked through to an internal temperature of 160°F, being careful not to overbake.

6. Slice the loaf into eight thick slices to serve.

PER SERVING Calories: 437; Fat: 34g; Protein: 28g; Total Carbs: 5g; Fiber: 1g; Net Carbs: 4g
70% fat, 26% protein, 4% carbs

PREP TIP: Use a muffin tin to make perfectly portioned servings. You'll want to eat a few to make a complete portion—for example, if you make 16 muffin-size loaves, 2 muffins would make a complete portion. You can easily freeze the remaining loaves for later meals. This recipe also works beautifully as meatballs with marinara sauce and Zucchini Noodles (page 220).

Ginger Pork Meatballs

Serves 4 / Prep time: 10 minutes / Cook time: 15 minutes

DAIRY FREE • NUT FREE • 30 MINUTES OR LESS

The spicy ginger and rich coconut flavors in these meatballs are a fun change of pace from the toothsome tomato-based classic. Serve them in lettuce cups, with Cauliflower Rice (page 218), or over Zucchini Noodles (page 220) with plenty of extra low-sodium soy sauce and lime juice.

1 egg, whisked

¼ cup almond flour

1 teaspoon minced ginger

1 teaspoon minced garlic

½ teaspoon sea salt

¼ teaspoon freshly ground
   black pepper

¼ cup minced cilantro

1 cup roughly chopped spinach

1 scallion, thinly sliced

1 pound ground pork

2 tablespoons coconut oil

1. Whisk the egg, almond flour, ginger, garlic, salt, and pepper in a large mixing bowl. Stir in the cilantro, spinach, and scallion.

2. Add the pork, and using your hands, mix the ingredients until combined. Shape the pork mixture into 8 to 12 meatballs.

3. Heat a large skillet over medium-high heat. Melt the coconut oil. When it is hot, sear the meatballs on all sides until well browned and cooked through to an internal temperature of 160°F, about 15 minutes.

PER SERVING Calories: 460; Fat: 35g; Protein: 33g; Total Carbs: 3g; Fiber: 1g; Net Carbs: 2g
68% fat, 29% protein, 3% carbs

PREP TIP: Form the meatballs ahead of time and allow them to rest uncovered in the refrigerator for up to 8 hours. This allows the flavors to come together and the exterior of the meatball to form a skin, which will help seal in all of the delicious juices.

Swedish Meatballs

Serves 4 / Prep time: 10 minutes / Cook time: 25 minutes

30 MINUTES OR LESS

If a certain big box superstore comes to mind when you think of Swedish meatballs, you're in for a treat. Sure, you can freeze them to enjoy later if you like, but they taste oh-so-good when prepared fresh, seared to perfection, and then simmered in a beef and wine reduction with butter and sour cream.

2 tablespoons canola oil, divided

1 cup minced onion

1 teaspoon minced garlic

1 egg, whisked

¼ cup almond flour

⅛ teaspoon ground allspice

¼ teaspoon ground nutmeg

½ teaspoon sea salt

½ teaspoon freshly ground
    black pepper

½ pound ground beef

½ pound ground pork

1 cup Beef Bone Broth (page 225)
    or low-sodium beef broth

¼ cup white wine

2 tablespoons cold butter

½ cup sour cream

1. Heat 1 tablespoon of the canola oil in a large skillet over medium heat. Add the onion and garlic and cook until soft, about 5 minutes.

2. In a mixing bowl, mix together the egg, almond flour, allspice, nutmeg, salt, and pepper. Add the beef, pork, and cooked onion mixture. Using your hands, mix the ingredients until combined. Form the mixture into 8 to 12 meatballs.

3. In the same skillet, heat the remaining tablespoon of canola oil and sear the meatballs on all sides until well browned and cooked through to an internal temperature of 160°F, about 15 minutes. Transfer the meatballs to a separate dish.

continued >

4. Deglaze the pan with the white wine, scraping up any browned bits from the bottom of the pan. Add the beef broth and bring to a simmer until reduced to about ½ cup of liquid.

5. Whisk in the butter until melted. Stir in the sour cream and return the meatballs to the pan. Simmer gently over low heat until the meatballs are heated through, about 2 minutes, or until ready to serve.

PER SERVING Calories: 509; Fat: 42g; Protein: 29g; Total Carbs: 3g; Fiber: 1g; Net Carbs: 1g
74% fat, 23% protein, 3% carbs

Rosemary Roasted Beef Tenderloin

Serves 4 / Prep time: 5 minutes / Cook time: 30 to 35 minutes

KETO QUOTIENT

1 ② 3

DAIRY FREE

The fragrant rosemary infuses the beef tenderloin with flavor as it cooks. Take your time browning the meat; it really does make a difference in the finished dish. The dish is versatile and goes beautifully with Pan-Roasted Brussels Sprouts with Bacon (page 112) or Creamed Broccoli (page 118).

1¼ pounds beef tenderloin

Sea salt

Freshly ground black pepper

2 sprigs fresh rosemary

1 tablespoon coconut oil

1. Preheat the oven to 350°F.

2. Heat a large cast iron or other ovenproof skillet over medium-high heat until hot, about 2 minutes.

3. While the pan heats, season the beef generously on all sides with salt and pepper. Place the rosemary sprigs on the beef and secure them with kitchen twine.

4. Add the oil to the skillet and tilt to coat the pan in the oil. Sear the tenderloin until it is browned on all sides, about 10 minutes.

5. Transfer the pan to the oven and finish roasting for 20 to 25 minutes until the beef is cooked through to an internal temperature of 145°F for medium-rare. For medium, cook an additional 3 to 5 minutes. For medium-well, cook an additional 8 to 10 minutes. Allow to rest for 10 minutes after you remove it from the oven.

PER SERVING Calories: 382; Fat: 30g; Protein: 28g; Total Carbs: 0g; Fiber: 0g; Net Carbs: 0g
71% fat, 29% protein, 4% carbs

VARIATION TIP: Sage makes a delicious alternative to rosemary.

Slow Cooker Pork Carnitas

**KETO
QUOTIENT**

1 2 3

Serves 4 / Prep time: 5 minutes / Cook time: 8 to 10 hours

DAIRY FREE • NUT FREE

*These pork Carnitas are delicious over Cauliflower Rice (page 218)
or served in lettuce leaves with a few slices of avocado and a dollop of
sour cream.*

1 tablespoon extra-virgin olive oil

1½ pounds boneless pork shoulder

2 teaspoons dried oregano

1 teaspoon ground cumin

⅛ teaspoon ground cloves

Zest and juice of 1 orange

Sea salt

Freshly ground black pepper

1 red onion, halved and sliced

4 garlic cloves, roughly chopped

1 cinnamon stick

1. Coat the interior of the slow cooker with the olive oil.

2. Season the pork with the oregano, cumin, cloves, orange zest, salt, and
   pepper. Place the pork in the slow cooker. Scatter the onion slices, garlic,
   and cinnamon stick around the pork. Sprinkle with the orange juice.

3. Cook on low for 8 to 10 hours, or until the meat is tender. Shred with two
   forks before serving.

PER SERVING Calories: 599; Fat: 44g; Protein: 41g; Total Carbs: 7g; Fiber: 1g; Net Carbs: 6g
68% fat, 27% protein, 5% carbs

Braised Beef Short Ribs

Serves 4 / Prep time: 10 minutes / Cook time: 2 hours, 15 minutes

DAIRY FREE • NUT FREE

Short ribs are a low-carb dieter's dream! The meat is succulent, flavorful, and loaded with fat. During an especially dark and stormy spring, I prepared these for my kids and myself, and we devoured them. They're awesome served over Celery Root Purée (page 116).

1 tablespoon coconut oil

4 beef short ribs, about 1½ pounds

Sea salt

Freshly ground pepper

2 carrots, diced

2 celery stalks, diced

1 onion, diced

2 garlic cloves, minced

4 ounces red wine

4 cups Beef Bone Broth (page 225)

1 tablespoon minced fresh oregano

2 tablespoons minced fresh parsley

1 scallion, minced

Zest of 1 lemon

2 packed cups leafy greens,
    such as lettuce

1. Preheat the oven to 325°F.

2. Heat a large cast iron or other ovenproof skillet over medium-high heat. Add the coconut oil. Pat the short ribs dry with paper towels. Season generously with salt and pepper.

3. When the oil is hot, season the short ribs liberally with salt and pepper. Sear them on all sides in the pan until well browned, about 10 minutes.

4. Deglaze the pan with the red wine, scraping up any browned bits. Add the carrots, celery, onion, garlic, and beef broth, and bring to a simmer. Return the short ribs to the pan, and cover with a lid. Transfer to the oven and bake for 2 hours, until the meat is meltingly tender.

5. While the meat cooks, in a small dish, mix together the oregano, parsley, scallion, and lemon zest. Set aside.

continued >

6. Transfer the vegetables to serving dishes. Carefully return the skillet to the stove and simmer the sauce over medium heat until reduced to about 1 cup of liquid, about 5 minutes.

7. Remove the bones from the short ribs and place the meat on top of the vegetables. Pour the pan sauce over the top.

8. Garnish with the fresh lettuce and the lemon herb mixture.

PER SERVING Calories: 774; Fat: 65g; Protein: 30g; Total Carbs: 10g; Fiber: 4g; Net Carbs: 6g
81% fat, 15% protein, 4% carbs

INGREDIENT TIP: Although fat and calories are not typically avoided on a ketogenic diet, the amount of beef fat in this dish may be difficult to digest and offer more calories than you need. To reduce the calories and fat in this dish, skim the fat from the surface of the pan before reducing the sauce.

BBQ Baby Back Ribs

Serves 4 / Prep time: 10 minutes / Cook time: 3 hours

DAIRY FREE • NUT FREE

KETO
QUOTIENT

1 ② 3

Slow roasting produces flavorful, succulent ribs that fall off the bone. I adapted this barbecue sauce recipe from one I found in Saveur *magazine. It was already low in carbs, but I omitted the sugar and used stevia, which worked perfectly. When combined with the pan juices from the pork ribs, it is pure awesome sauce!*

2 teaspoons smoked paprika

¾ teaspoon ground cumin

1 teaspoon onion powder

1 teaspoon garlic powder

1½-pound rack of pork ribs

Sea salt

Freshly ground black pepper

½ cup apple cider vinegar

2 tablespoons ketchup

2 to 3 drops liquid stevia

¼ cup minced cilantro

1 scallion, roughly chopped

1. Preheat the oven to 250°F.

2. Mix the paprika, cumin, onion powder, and garlic powder in a small mixing bowl.

3. Season the ribs with salt and pepper and half of the spice blend. Place the ribs into a roasting pan or Dutch oven fitted with a lid. Alternatively, cover the baking dish tightly with foil. Bake for 2½ hours.

4. While the ribs cook, mix together the vinegar, ketchup, and the remaining spice blend in a small saucepan over medium heat. Simmer for 10 minutes, until reduced slightly. Sweeten with a few drops of liquid stevia. Transfer the barbecue sauce to a blender along with the cilantro and scallion.

5. Remove the pork from the oven and transfer the cooked ribs to a separate dish momentarily.

continued >

6. Carefully remove ½ cup of the accumulated pan juices from the roasting pan. Add it to the blender and purée until smooth.

7. Discard the remaining pan juices and then return the ribs to the pan. Pour the barbecue sauce over the ribs and roast uncovered for 30 minutes.

PER SERVING Calories: 654; Fat: 51g; Protein: 42g; Total Carbs: 6g; Fiber: 1g; Net Carbs: 5g
70% fat, 26% protein, 4% carbs

INGREDIENT TIP: To reduce the carbs even further, look for a reduced-sugar ketch-up and always avoid brands that contain high-fructose corn syrup.

Roasted Pork Belly and Asparagus

Serves 4 / Prep time: 5 minutes / Cook time: 2 hours, 45 minutes

DAIRY FREE • NUT FREE

Pork belly is inexpensive and renders its fat to produce a deliciously crispy exterior and tender, succulent meat. Setting the meat on a rack allows the fat to drip into the pan below. You can roast any non-starchy vegetable in the fat. I am partial to asparagus, but fennel, carrots, egg-plant, or red onions would also be lovely.

2½ pounds pork belly

1 tablespoon canola oil

Sea salt

Freshly ground black pepper

1 pound asparagus,
    woody stems removed

1. Preheat the oven to 325°F. Place an oven-safe rack inside a roasting pan.

2. Place the pork skin-side up on the rack and coat with the oil. Season liberally with salt. Roast uncovered for 2 hours.

3. Increase the heat to 400°F and cook the pork for another 30 minutes to crisp up the skin. Carefully transfer the pork to a cutting board to rest. Remove the rack from the pan.

4. Scatter the asparagus in the roasting pan in the rendered pork fat. Season with salt and pepper. Roast for 15 minutes until crisp tender. Transfer to a serving platter. Slice the pork belly into four equal portions and serve with the roasted asparagus.

PER SERVING Calories: 616; Fat: 60g; Protein: 13g; Total Carbs: 6g; Fiber: 3g; Net Carbs: 3g
87% fat, 8% protein, 5% carbs

Lemongrass Pork Noodle Bowls

Serves 4 / Prep time: 10 minutes / Cook time: 30 minutes

DAIRY FREE • NUT FREE

The pungent flavors of serrano pepper, lemongrass, and garlic permeate these flavorful noodle bowls. They have all the flavor and a fraction of the carbs of the traditional Vietnamese dish.

1 tablespoon minced lemongrass	1¼-pound pork tenderloin
1 serrano pepper, minced	2 zucchini
2 teaspoons minced garlic	2 carrots
2 tablespoons low-sodium soy sauce	½ cup fresh basil leaves
2 tablespoons lime juice	½ cup fresh cilantro
¼ cup canola oil	½ cup fresh mint leaves

1. Preheat the oven to 400°F. Line a baking dish with parchment paper.

2. In a glass measuring cup, whisk together the lemongrass, chile, garlic, soy sauce, lime juice, and oil. Pour half of the mixture over the pork tenderloin, turning to coat.

3. Place the pork in the baking dish and roast for 30 minutes, or until cooked to an internal temperature of 145°F. Set aside on a cutting board to rest.

4. While the pork cooks, run the zucchini and carrots through a spiralizer. If you don't have a spiralizer, use a vegetable peeler to cut the vegetables into long, flat noodles. Place the noodles in a large salad bowl and toss them with the remaining dressing.

5. Just before serving, toss the noodles with the basil, cilantro, and mint, and then divide among the serving bowls. Thinly slice the pork tenderloin and place equal portions on top of each noodle serving.

PER SERVING Calories: 446; Fat: 25g; Protein: 44g; Total Carbs: 9g; Fiber: 3g; Net Carbs: 6g
50% fat, 39% protein, 11% carbs

PREP TIP: Make the dressing ahead of time and let the pork marinate for up to 8 hours covered in the refrigerator before roasting.

Beef Bourguignon

KETO
QUOTIENT

1 (2) 3

Serves 4 / Prep time: 10 minutes / Cook time: 2 hours

NUT FREE

I learned to make beef bourguignon while living in Europe, where I was obsessed with French food. When I was asked to prepare dinner for 70 guests, including a visiting dignitary, I knew this classic dish had to be on the menu. Don't forget to whisk the cold butter in at the end; it really makes the sauce.

1 tablespoon canola oil

1½ pounds beef chuck, cut into
   2-inch cubes

Sea salt

Freshly ground black pepper

¼ cup cognac (optional)

3 cups dry red wine

1 cup Beef Bone Broth (page 225)
   or low-sodium beef stock

1 cup cremini mushrooms, halved

1 cup pearl onions, blanched and
   skins removed

1 sprig fresh rosemary

1 sprig fresh thyme

1 garlic clove, smashed

2 tablespoons cold butter

1. Preheat the oven to 325°F.

2. Heat the canola oil in a large Dutch oven over medium-high heat.

3. Pat the beef cubes dry with paper towels, and season generously with salt and pepper. Working in batches to avoid crowding the pan, brown the beef cubes on all sides, about 5 minutes per batch. Transfer the seared beef to a separate plate.

4. When all the meat has browned, carefully pour the cognac (if using) into the pot. If the pot is very hot, it may ignite, so avert your face. Cook for 1 minute to burn off some of the alcohol.

5. Add the red wine and beef broth and bring to simmer, scraping up the browned bits from the bottom of the pan. Return the seared beef and any accumulated juices to the pan along with the mushrooms, onions, rosemary, thyme, and garlic. Cover the pot and transfer to the oven. Cook for 1½ hours, or until the meat is very tender.

6. Carefully return the pot to the stove and transfer the meat and vegetables to a serving platter. Simmer the cooking liquid over medium heat until reduced to only 1 cup of liquid, about 10 minutes. Whisk in the cold butter 1 tablespoon at a time.

7. Pour the sauce over the meat and vegetables and serve.

PER SERVING Calories: 657; Fat: 40g; Protein: 33g; Total Carbs: 10g; Fiber: 1g; Net Carbs: 9g 75% fat, 20% protein, 5% carbs

PREP TIP: To save time and money, purchase frozen pearl onions, which have already been blanched and peeled.

Beef Mushroom Stroganoff

Serves 4 / Prep time: 10 minutes / Cook time: 15 minutes

NUT FREE • 30 MINUTES OR LESS

Who says stroganoff has to include pasta? Only Americans, it turns out. The traditional Russian dish is usually served with pickles and mashed potatoes. So whip up a batch of Mashed Cauliflower (page 219) and call it good. My friend Christine made this stroganoff for Christmas Eve dinner, and I was hooked! Her secret: demi-glace. Purchase a small container of this flavor gold mine at a well-stocked grocery store, order online, or make your own with the tip below.

1 tablespoon canola oil

1¼ pounds well-marbled rib-eye steak, thinly sliced on an angle

Sea salt

Freshly ground black pepper

1 yellow onion, halved and thinly sliced

8 ounces cremini mushrooms, sliced

¼ cup brandy

½ cup Beef Bone Broth (page 225) or water

2 tablespoons demi-glace

1 bay leaf

1 teaspoon whole-grain mustard

1 cup sour cream

2 tablespoons roughly chopped parsley

1. Heat the canola oil in a large skillet over medium-high heat.

2. Season the steak with salt and pepper and sear until just cooked through, about 3 minutes. Transfer the steak to a separate plate.

3. Cook the onion and mushrooms in the same skillet until tender, about 7 minutes.

4. Add the brandy and deglaze the pan, scraping up the browned bits.

5. Return the steak along with any accumulated juices to the pan along with the broth, demi-glace, bay leaf, and mustard, and simmer for 5 minutes. Remove the pan from the heat, remove the bay leaf, and stir in the sour cream. Sprinkle with fresh parsley to serve.

PER SERVING Calories: 605; Fat: 47g; Protein: 30g; Total Carbs: 7g; Fiber: 1g; Net Carbs: 6g
73% fat, 22% protein, 5% carbs

INGREDIENT TIP: To make your own demi-glace, mix together 1 quart of beef broth with 1 cup of red wine and 1 tablespoon of tomato paste. Simmer over low heat until reduced to about 1 cup. This will take several hours.

Lamb Meatball Salad with Yogurt Dressing

Serves 4 / Prep time: 10 minutes / Cook time: 20 minutes

30 MINUTES OR LESS

This hearty Greek salad platter is perfect for sharing and has an appealing balance of flavors and textures—creamy, cooling yogurt sauce, savory lamb meatballs, briny olives, and smoky roasted red peppers. Making the meatballs and the sauce ahead of time allows the flavors to come together.

¼ cup almond flour

¼ cup minced red onion

1 teaspoon minced garlic

1 egg, whisked

2 tablespoons minced fresh parsley

1 tablespoon minced fresh oregano

½ teaspoon sea salt, plus more
   for seasoning

½ teaspoon freshly ground
   black pepper, plus more
   for seasoning

1 pound ground lamb

½ cup plain whole-milk yogurt

¼ cup full-fat mayonnaise

1 teaspoon minced fresh dill

1 teaspoon minced fresh garlic

1 cup fresh mint leaves

2 cups baby spinach

4 cups hand-torn romaine lettuce

4 roasted red bell peppers,
   sliced into 2-inch pieces

½ cup diced peeled cucumbers

½ cup assorted pitted olives

1. Preheat the oven to 400°F.

2. In a mixing bowl, mix together the almond flour, onion, garlic, egg, parsley, oregano, ½ teaspoon salt, and ½ teaspoon pepper.

3. Add the lamb to the bowl, and using your hands, mix the ingredients until combined. Shape the mixture into 16 small meatballs.

4. Place the meatballs on a rimmed baking sheet and bake for 20 minutes, or until gently browned and cooked through.

5. While the meatballs bake, make the yogurt dressing. In a small bowl, mix the yogurt, mayonnaise, dill, and garlic. Season to taste with salt and pepper.

6. To serve, place the mint, spinach, lettuce, bell peppers, cucumbers, and olives on a large serving platter. Top with the cooked lamb meatballs and pour the yogurt dressing over the salad. Season with more freshly ground pepper.

PER SERVING Calories: 568; Fat: 47g; Protein: 26g; Total Carbs: 11g; Fiber: 3g; Net Carbs: 8g
74% fat, 18% protein, 8% carbs

INGREDIENT TIP: To save money on fresh herbs, look for herb blends, which usually contain three different herbs. They are sold with the other fresh herbs in the produce section.

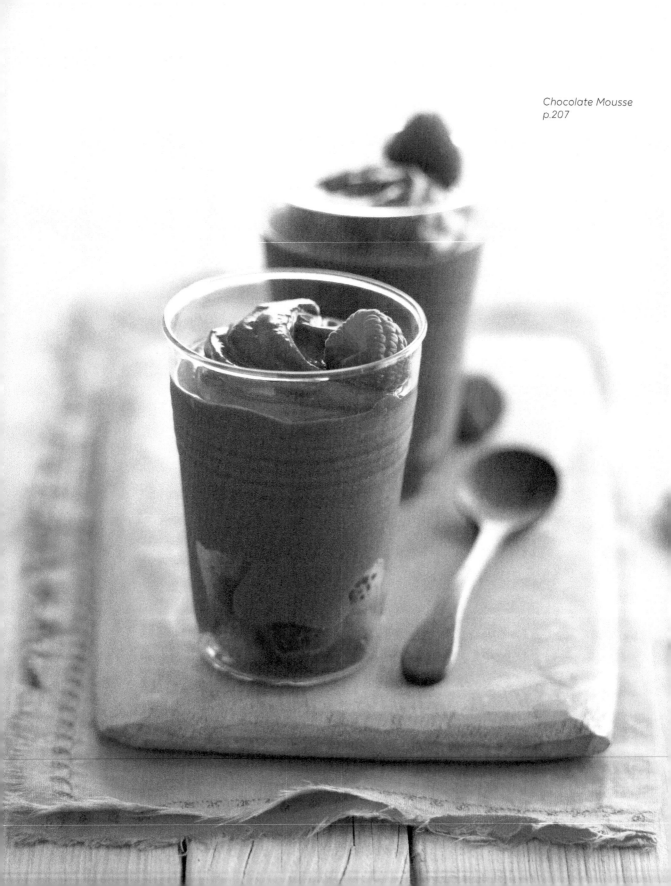

*Chocolate Mousse
p.207*

CHAPTER ELEVEN

Desserts

Key Lime Pie Fat Bombs

Serves 16 / Prep time: 5 minutes, plus 15 minutes to chill / Cook time: 0 minutes

VEGETARIAN • 30 MINUTES OR LESS

These fat bombs are like miniature slices of key lime pie. They're sweet, tangy, and creamy in the center and coated with a macadamia nut and coconut crust.

8 ounces cream cheese

2 teaspoons lime zest

2 tablespoons lime juice

¼ teaspoon liquid stevia

½ cup shredded unsweetened coconut, finely ground

½ cup macadamia nuts, finely ground

¼ teaspoon sea salt

1. In a bowl, mix together the cream cheese, lime zest, lime juice, and liquid stevia.

2. In a shallow dish, mix together the coconut, macadamia nuts, and sea salt.

3. Divide the cream cheese mixture into 16 small balls, about 1 tablespoon each. Roll the balls in the coconut mixture.

4. Place the balls in a covered container and refrigerate for at least 15 minutes before serving. The fat bombs will keep for up to one week in the refrigerator or up to one month in the freezer.

PER SERVING Calories: 98; Fat: 10g; Protein: 2g; Total Carbs: 3g; Fiber: 1g; Net Carbs: 2g
96% fat, 2% protein, 2% carbs

PREP TIP: Process the coconut and macadamia nuts in a food processor or a clean coffee grinder until they are finely ground.

No-Bake Coconut Chocolate Squares

Serves 24 / Prep time: 10 minutes, plus 45 minutes to chill / Cook time: 0 minutes

VEGETARIAN • DAIRY FREE • NUT FREE

KETO QUOTIENT

1 2 ③

These sweet squares are a delicious dessert or yummy snack. The coconut oil helps keep you in ketosis, while the chocolate satisfies your chocolate cravings.

1½ cups coconut oil, at room temperature, divided

1 cup shredded unsweetened coconut

¼ teaspoon liquid stevia, divided

½ cup unsweetened cocoa powder

½ teaspoon vanilla extract

⅛ teaspoon sea salt

1. Line an 8-by-8-inch baking dish with parchment paper.

2. In a bowl, mix together 1 cup of the coconut oil with the unsweetened coconut, and ⅛ teaspoon of liquid stevia. Spread the mixture in the baking dish and smooth it down with a spatula. Place it in the freezer for 15 minutes to set.

3. Melt the remaining ½ cup of coconut oil in a glass measuring cup. Whisk in the cocoa powder, vanilla extract, sea salt, and remaining ⅛ teaspoon of stevia. Pour the chocolate mixture over the chilled coconut layer.

4. Place the dish in the refrigerator and allow to set for 30 minutes. Slice into 24 squares.

PER SERVING (1 square) Calories: 144; Fat: 16g; Protein: 1g; Total Carbs: 2g; Fiber: 1g; Net Carbs: 1g; 98% fat, 1% protein, 1% carbs

VARIATION TIP: Sprinkle the top of these coconut chocolate squares with ½ cup toasted, roughly chopped pecans for added texture and flavor.

VARIATION PER SERVING Calories: 161; Fat: 17g; Protein: 1g; Total Carbs: 2g; Fiber: 1g; Net Carbs: 1g; 98% fat, 1% protein, 1% carbs

Chocolate Chip Cookies

Serves 16 / Prep time: 10 minutes / Cook time: 20 minutes

VEGETARIAN • 30 MINUTES OR LESS

Chocolate chip cookies are my undoing. Since going gluten-free five years ago, I rarely find myself tempted because I can't even have a crumb! But then these gluten-free, low-carb chocolate chip cookies emerge from the oven, and I'm in heaven. These cookies don't have the same effect on blood sugar and insulin production, so they won't trigger excessive cravings.

2 cups almond flour

½ cup Swerve or another
   non-caloric sweetener

1 teaspoon baking powder

½ teaspoon sea salt

3 tablespoons butter

2 tablespoons milk

1 tablespoon vanilla extract

½ cup dark chocolate chips,
   at least 60 percent cacao

½ cup roughly chopped pecans

1. Preheat the oven to 350°F. Line a baking sheet with parchment paper.

2. In a mixing bowl, mix together the almond flour, Swerve, baking powder, and sea salt.

3. Add the butter, milk, and vanilla, and stir to mix. Fold in the chocolate chips and pecans.

4. Using half of the mixture, form 8 equal-size cookies on the baking sheet. Flatten each gently with the palm of your hand. Bake for 10 minutes, or until barely golden brown around the edges. Transfer to a cooling rack and repeat with the remaining cookie dough, making another 8 cookies.

PER SERVING (1 cookie) Calories: 144; Fat: 13g; Protein: 4g; Total Carbs: 6g; Fiber: 2g; Net Carbs: 4g; 75% fat, 10% protein, 15% carbs

PREP TIP: I like to divide the batch in half and shape the second half into a long cylinder, wrap in parchment or plastic wrap, and place in the freezer. Then they're available for baking whenever the mood strikes.

Peanut Butter Cookies

Serves 30 / Prep time: 10 minutes / Cook time: 30 minutes

VEGETARIAN

I remember baking peanut butter cookies as a child and carefully dipping a fork into granulated sugar to make perfect impressions on the surface of each cookie. This version has a fraction of the carbs of those childhood treats but still brings back all of the happy memories with my mom in the kitchen.

¾ cup butter, at room temperature

1 cup plus 2 tablespoons Swerve
  or another non-caloric sweetener

1 cup natural peanut butter

2 eggs

1 teaspoon vanilla extract

2 cups almond flour

2 tablespoons coconut flour

1 teaspoon sea salt

1 teaspoon baking soda

1. Preheat the oven to 350°F. Line a baking sheet with parchment paper.

2. In a large mixing bowl, beat the butter and Swerve together until light and fluffy, about 1 minute.

3. Add the peanut butter, eggs, and vanilla extract, and beat until fully emulsified, another minute.

4. Stir in the almond flour, coconut flour, sea salt, and baking soda.

5. Using one-third of the mixture, form 10 equal-size cookies on the baking sheet. Flatten each cookie with the back of a fork that has been dipped in Swerve.

6. Bake for 10 minutes, or until barely golden brown around the edges. Transfer to a cooling rack and repeat with the remaining cookie dough, making another 20 cookies total.

PER SERVING (1 cookie) Calories: 146; Fat: 13g; Protein: 4g; Total Carbs: 4g; Fiber: 2g; Net Carbs: 2g; 80% fat, 10% protein, 10% carbs

SUBSTITUTION TIP: These cookies can also be made with almond butter if you are sensitive to peanuts.

Cream Cheese Pound Cake

Serves 12 / Prep time: 10 minutes / Cook time: 40 to 45 minutes

VEGETARIAN

I typically use liquid stevia as a sugar substitute, but in cakes and certain other baked goods, sugar adds structure and moisture. For this pound cake, Swerve, made with the sugar alcohol erythritol, is a good alternative. It has no effect on blood sugar, and for many, there's less of the digestive distress caused by other sugar alcohols such as xylitol.

4 ounces butter, at room temperature

8 ounces cream cheese, at room temperature

1¼ cups Swerve or another non-caloric sweetener

6 eggs

1 tablespoon vanilla extract

2 cups almond flour

⅓ cup coconut flour

1 tablespoon aluminum-free double-acting baking powder

½ teaspoon sea salt

1. Preheat the oven to 350°F. Line a 9-by-13-inch loaf pan with parchment paper.

2. Beat the butter, cream cheese, and Swerve with a hand mixer until smooth and creamy, about 1 minute. Add the eggs and vanilla extract, and beat until thoroughly emulsified.

3. Stir in the almond flour, coconut flour, baking powder, and sea salt. Mix until just combined. Pour into the prepared pan.

4. Bake for 40 to 45 minutes, or until a toothpick inserted into the center comes out clean.

PER SERVING Calories: 288; Fat: 26g; Protein: 9g; Total Carbs: 7g; Fiber: 3g; Net Carbs: 4g 81% fat, 13% protein, 6% carbs

VARIATION TIP: Stir in 1 tablespoon of minced fresh rosemary for a more complex cake.

Chocolate Mousse

Serves 4 / Prep time: 10 minutes / Cook time: 0 minutes

NUT FREE • 30 MINUTES OR LESS

*I didn't learn to love chocolate mousse until I learned to make it myself.
At restaurants, it was always too fluffy, like chocolate air. I prefer a
thicker mousse that borders on pudding. This can also be spread into
a baking dish or ice pop molds and frozen.*

3 ounces dark chocolate,
   85 percent cacao

4 eggs, separated

Pinch sea salt

1 teaspoon vanilla extract

½ cup heavy cream

1 teaspoon liquid stevia

½ cup raspberries (optional)

1. In a heavy-bottomed saucepan over low heat, or in a double boiler over
   a pot of barely simmering water, heat the chocolate for about 5 minutes
   until melted. Set aside to cool.

2. In a medium mixing bowl, combine the egg whites and salt. Beat the eggs
   until stiff peaks form, about 3 minutes. Set aside.

3. In a separate mixing bowl, beat the heavy cream and stevia until thick,
   about 3 minutes.

4. Stir the egg yolks and vanilla into the cooled, melted chocolate.

5. Add a generous spoonful of the whipped egg whites and whipped cream
   to the chocolate, and mix well.

6. Transfer the chocolate mixture and the whipped cream to the bowl with
   the egg whites and fold gently until combined.

continued >

7. Divide the mousse among the serving cups. Top with raspberries, if desired.

PER SERVING Calories: 288; Fat: 26g; Protein: 9g; Total Carbs: 6g; Fiber: 1g; Net Carbs: 5g
81% fat, 12% protein, 7% carbs

INGREDIENT TIP: Choose good-quality dark chocolate for this mousse. I usually opt for chocolate from the brands Green & Black's, Scharffen Berger, or Alter Eco. The extra-dark varieties with greater than 70 percent cacao often have as few as 2 grams of carbohydrates per square, making them a delicious treat on a low-carb diet.

Ice Cream

Serves 16 / Prep time: 5 minutes, plus 4 hours chilling time / Cook time: 10 minutes

NUT FREE

This essential ice cream recipe can be taken in any direction you desire. I make ice cream more often than anyone really should. The variations are endless, and I love being able to control how much sweetener I add. Now, when I taste commercial varieties, they are far too sweet.

2 cups heavy cream

2 cups whole milk

4 egg yolks

Pinch sea salt

1 tablespoon vanilla extract

1 teaspoon liquid stevia

1. In a saucepan over low heat, whisk together the cream, milk, egg yolks, and salt until the eggs are thoroughly incorporated.

2. Cook, stirring often until the mixture thickens and coats the back of a spoon, about 10 minutes, being careful not to heat over 150°F.

3. Stir in the vanilla extract and stevia, adding more stevia to taste, if desired. Pour this mixture through a strainer into a separate dish and cover with parchment paper or plastic wrap to prevent skin from forming on the surface. Refrigerate until thoroughly chilled, about 4 hours.

4. Transfer the mixture to an ice cream maker and freeze according to the manufacturer's instructions.

PER SERVING (½ cup) Calories: 135; Fat: 13g; Protein: 2g; Total Carbs: 2g; Fiber: 0g; Net Carbs: 2g; 88% fat, 6% protein, 6% carbs

SUBSTITUTION TIP: To make this ice cream dairy free, swap the heavy cream and milk for 1¾ cups (1 can) of coconut cream and 2 cups of almond milk.

PREP TIP: If you do not have an ice cream maker, place a large ceramic baking dish into the freezer for 2 hours. Pour the chilled ice cream base into the dish and return it to the freezer. Stir the ice cream with a spatula every 30 minutes until it is frozen and thick, about 2 hours.

Sangria Granita

KETO
QUOTIENT

1 2 3

Serves 8 / Prep time: 5 minutes / Cook time: 5 minutes

DAIRY FREE • NUT FREE • VEGETARIAN • 30 MINUTES OR LESS

Sangria is a traditional Spanish chilled wine and fruit drink often served with tapas. This version has the cinnamon and orange flavors of the original, but it omits the additional fruit and added sugar for a much lower carb version. While some of the alcohol cooks off, it is definitely a grown-up dessert!

1 bottle fruity red wine,
   such as Tempranillo or Rioja

3 ounces brandy

1 cinnamon stick

Zest and juice of 1 orange

1 teaspoon liquid stevia

1. In a medium saucepan, mix together the wine, brandy, cinnamon stick, and orange zest and juice. Bring to a gentle simmer for 2 minutes, then allow the mixture to steep for 10 minutes. Stir in the liquid stevia.

2. Pour the mixture through a sieve into a shallow glass baking dish and transfer it to the freezer. Freeze until solid, about 2 hours.

3. Using the tines of a fork, rake through the frozen sangria to produce fine crystals. Divide the granita among the chilled serving glasses. Store leftovers in a covered container in the freezer.

PER SERVING Calories: 102; Fat: 0g; Protein: 0g; Total Carbs: 3g; Fiber: 0g; Net Carbs: 3g
0% fat, 0% protein, 12% carbs (remaining calories are from alcohol)

New York Cheesecake

Serves 16 / Prep time: 15 minutes / Cook time: 1 hour, 15 minutes

VEGETARIAN

A cheesecake is a labor of love, but its rich, creamy texture and sweet vanilla flavor are worth the effort. Cheesecake is naturally a great fit for low-carb baking because the cream cheese, eggs, and heavy cream are the essential ingredients, and they remain unchanged. This recipe uses ground hazelnuts for the crust, which have a surprisingly similar texture to traditional graham cracker crusts.

2 cups hazelnuts

1½ cups plus 1 tablespoon Swerve
    or equivalent non-caloric
    sweetener, divided

1 teaspoon sea salt

2 tablespoons butter, melted

32 ounces cream cheese,
    at room temperature

1 tablespoon vanilla extract

2 eggs

¾ cup heavy cream

1. Preheat the oven to 350°F.

2. In a food processor, pulse the hazelnuts, 1 tablespoon of Swerve, and sea salt until the hazelnuts are finely ground. Drizzle the butter into the hazelnuts, and pulse a few times until just combined.

3. Spread the hazelnut mixture in the bottom of a 9-inch springform pan. Press down with the back of a fork, coming up the sides by about ½ inch. Bake for 10 minutes. Transfer to a cooling rack.

4. When cool, wrap the pan with a large sheet of aluminum foil to prevent water from seeping into the pan later.

5. While the crust cools, prepare the filling. In a large mixing bowl, beat together half of the remaining Swerve and half of the cream cheese until smooth and fluffy, about 2 minutes. Add the remaining Swerve and cream cheese, and beat for another minute. Add the vanilla, then the eggs one at a time, beating thoroughly after each addition. Add in the heavy cream, and beat until just combined.

continued >

6. Pour the mixture into the prepared crust. Transfer the pan to a larger roasting dish and pour water into it until it comes halfway up the sides of the cheesecake pan.

7. Bake for 1 hour and 15 minutes, or until the cheesecake is almost completely set. The center will still be slightly wobbly. Remove from the water bath and allow to cool for 1 hour, then refrigerate until ready to serve.

PER SERVING Calories: 360; Fat: 36g; Protein: 8g; Total Carbs: 6g; Fiber: 2g; Net Carbs: 4g
85% fat, 8% protein, 7% carbs

SUBSTITUTION TIP: If you prefer to bake with liquid stevia instead of Swerve, use 1 teaspoon. The cake will be denser and shorter but equally delicious.

Crustless Cannoli

NUT FREE • 30 MINUTES OR LESS

KETO
QUOTIENT

1 **2** 3

I adore cannoli so much I even bought my own cannoli molds so I could make the crispy shells at home. That was before I stopped eating wheat and other grains. Bummer! Fortunately, the cannoli filling is pretty darn good on its own. And it's so much easier to make!

2 cups whole-milk ricotta cheese

1 teaspoon liquid stevia

1 teaspoon ground cinnamon

¼ teaspoon allspice

¼ teaspoon lemon zest

⅓ cup heavy cream

1 ounce grated dark chocolate

1. In a medium mixing bowl, stir together the ricotta, stevia, cinnamon, allspice, and lemon zest.

2. In a separate bowl, beat the heavy cream until thick and fluffy. Fold the heavy cream and grated chocolate into the ricotta mixture. Divide the mixture among the serving cups.

PER SERVING Calories: 268; Fat: 23g; Protein: 12g; Total Carbs: 5g; Fiber: 0g; Net Carbs: 5g
77% fat, 18% protein, 5% carbs

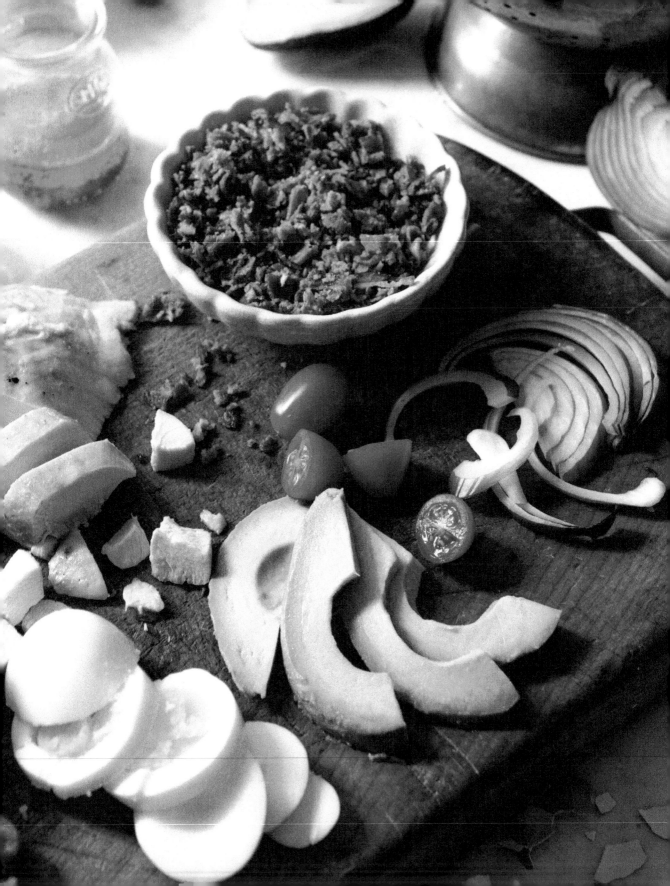

CHAPTER TWELVE
Staples

Cloud Bread

Serves 4 / Prep time: 10 minutes / Cook time: 25 to 30 minutes

NUT FREE • VEGETARIAN

These puffy little flatbreads are perfect for toasting, spreading with nut butter, or using for a sandwich. While I can't argue that they have the texture of traditional grain breads, they offer some of the convenience and comfort of bread.

3 eggs, separated

¼ teaspoon cream of tartar

Sea salt

3 tablespoons cream cheese

1 to 2 drops liquid stevia

1. Preheat the oven to 300°F. Line a rimmed baking sheet with parchment paper.

2. In a large mixing bowl, whip the egg whites, cream of tartar, and sea salt until stiff peaks form.

3. In a separate bowl, beat the egg yolks, cream cheese, and stevia until smooth.

4. Fold some of the egg white mixture into the egg yolk mixture, and then add the remaining egg white mixture.

5. Spoon the mixture into 8 mounds on the parchment paper, spreading each one out until it is about 3 inches wide.

6. Bake for 25 to 30 minutes or until the breads are dry and beginning to brown.

PER SERVING (2 pieces) Calories: 82; Fat: 6g; Protein: 6g; Total Carbs: 0g; Fiber: 0g; Net Carbs: 0g; 70% fat, 30% protein, 0% carbs

PREP TIP: Use a drinking glass to draw eight 3-inch circles with pencil on the parchment so that each cloud bread is identical in shape.

Bulletproof Coffee

Serves 1 / Prep time: 1 minute / Cook time: 0 minutes

NUT FREE • VEGETARIAN • 30 MINUTES OR LESS

This creamy beverage is a delicious way to start your day and gives you a generous dose of ketones right from the start. You don't have to have an immersion blender, but it sure helps, and it keeps the coffee from cooling off too quickly in a traditional blender.

8 ounces brewed hot coffee

1 tablespoon butter

1 tablespoon coconut oil

Combine all of the ingredients in a large mug. Place an immersion blender all the way into the cup. Pulse a few times until the brew is thick and frothy. Enjoy immediately.

PER SERVING Calories: 219; Fat: 25g; Protein: 0g; Total Carbs: 0g; Fiber: 0g; Net Carbs: 0g
100% fat, 0% protein, 0% carbs

INGREDIENT TIP: Choose butter from grass-fed cows for the best flavor and nutrition. Compared with butter from grain-fed cows, it is higher in omega-3 fatty acids and vitamin K_2.

Cauliflower Rice

Serves 4 / Prep time: 5 minutes / Cook time: 5 minutes

DAIRY FREE • NUT FREE • VEGETARIAN • 30 MINUTES OR LESS

The ratio of fat to carbs might not look like something you would find on a ketogenic diet, but this basic cauliflower rice is designed to accompany items much higher in fat and protein. One of the reasons it's so awesome on a low-carb diet is that it is versatile enough to go with a variety of foods and adds volume to an otherwise calorie-dense (small portions) diet.

1 large head of cauliflower, broken into florets

1 tablespoon coconut oil

Sea salt

1. Pulse the cauliflower in a food processor until coarsely ground, about the texture of rice.

2. Squeeze the cauliflower by the handful over the sink to remove excess moisture.

3. Heat the coconut oil in a large skillet over medium-high heat and stir-fry the cauliflower for 5 minutes, until just heated through. Season with salt.

PER SERVING Calories: 82; Fat: 4g; Protein: 4g; Total Carbs: 11g; Fiber: 5g; Net Carbs: 6g
44% fat, 20% protein, 36% carbs

Mashed Cauliflower

Serves 4 / Prep time: 5 minutes / Cook time: 10 minutes

NUT FREE • VEGETARIAN • 30 MINUTES OR LESS

KETO QUOTIENT

1 **2** 3

This mashed cauliflower has all of the creaminess of mashed potatoes with a fraction of the carbs. Serve it wherever you would normally enjoy mashed potatoes, such as with Braised Beef Short Ribs (page 187) or Roasted Pork Belly and Asparagus (page 191).

1 large head cauliflower, broken into florets

¼ cup heavy cream

2 tablespoons butter

Sea salt

1. Fill a large pot with 1 inch of water and add a steamer basket.

2. Place the cauliflower in the basket, cover the pot, and bring the water to a simmer. Cook for 10 minutes, or until the cauliflower is very tender.

3. Transfer the steamed cauliflower to a food processor along with the heavy cream, butter, and a generous pinch of sea salt. Purée until very smooth.

PER SERVING Calories: 155; Fat: 12g; Protein: 5g; Total Carbs: 11g; Fiber: 5g; Net Carbs: 6g
70% fat, 13% protein, 17% carbs

PREP TIP: If you do not have a steamer basket, simply place the cauliflower directly in the water and drain thoroughly in a colander before transferring to the food processor.

Zucchini Noodles

Serves 4 / Prep time: 5 minutes, plus 20 minutes inactive time
Cook time: 2 to 3 minutes

DAIRY FREE • NUT FREE • VEGETARIAN • 30 MINUTES OR LESS

Zucchini noodles, also called "zoodles," are another low-carb diet staple. They can be served raw in salads, but the texture is closer to traditional pasta if they are first salted to remove excess moisture and then sautéed quickly.

2 medium zucchini   2 tablespoons coconut oil
Sea salt

1. Cut off the stem ends of the zucchini. Place the cut side on the spiralizer blade and firmly attach the spiky end of the spiralizer to the opposite end of the zucchini. Run the zucchini through the spiralizer to produce long, thin noodles.

2. Place the zucchini noodles in a colander and season very generously with salt. Place the colander into the sink and let the zucchini sweat for 20 minutes.

3. Rinse the zucchini with fresh water and wring as much moisture as you can from the noodles, trying not to break them.

4. Heat a large skillet over high heat. When it is hot, add the coconut oil. When the oil is hot, sauté the zucchini noodles for 2 to 3 minutes, or until hot but not browned.

PER SERVING Calories: 75; Fat: 7g; Protein: 1g; Total Carbs: 4g; Fiber: 1g; Net Carbs: 3g
84% fat, 5% protein, 11% carbs

PREP TIP: If you do not have a spiralizer, use a vegetable peeler to produce a wide, flat noodle, more akin to fettuccine. You will have to discard sections toward the center of the zucchini that are filled with seeds.

Guacamole

Yields about 1⅓ cups / Prep time: 5 minutes / Cook time: 0 minutes

DAIRY FREE • NUT FREE • VEGETARIAN • 30 MINUTES OR LESS

If you're accustomed to a low-fat diet, you know that guacamole is kryptonite. With a whopping 20 grams of fat per serving, it's off-limits or the portion sizes are so small, why bother? Hooray for a high-fat diet— guacamole is back on the menu! Serve this alongside Carne Asada Chicken Bowls (page 158).

2 large avocados, pitted and peeled

2 tablespoons extra-virgin olive oil

¼ teaspoon sea salt

Juice of 1 lime

1 jalapeño pepper, ribs and seeds removed, minced

1 garlic clove, minced

1 small shallot, minced

1. Mash the avocado, olive oil, salt, and lime juice in a bowl, or use a mortar and pestle.

2. Fold in the pepper, garlic, and shallot. Serve immediately.

PER SERVING (about ⅓ cup per serving) Calories: 212; Fat: 20g; Protein: 2g; Total Carbs: 10g; Fiber: 6g; Net Carbs: 4g; 84% fat, 2% protein, 14% carbs

PREP TIP: Store any extra guacamole in the refrigerator. To keep it from turning brown, drizzle the top with extra lime juice and lay a piece of parchment paper or plastic wrap directly on the surface of the guacamole. Store in the refrigerator for up to two days.

Zucchini Hummus

Serves 4 / Prep time: 5 minutes / Cook time: 0 minutes

DAIRY FREE • NUT FREE • VEGETARIAN • 30 MINUTES OR LESS

Hummus and vegetables are my go-to snack, but the carbs add up quickly when you're using chickpeas. Zucchini is a surprising alternative that yields a similar flavor and texture. Just make sure to peel the zucchini; otherwise, you'll end up with green flecks in your hummus.

1 medium zucchini, peeled and diced

1 garlic clove

2 tablespoons lemon juice

¼ cup tahini

3 tablespoons extra-virgin olive oil

½ teaspoon sea salt

In a blender, purée the zucchini, garlic, lemon juice, tahini, olive oil, and sea salt until very smooth. Store in a covered container for up to three days.

PER SERVING Calories: 190; Fat: 18g; Protein: 3g; Total Carbs: 6g; Fiber: 2g; Net Carbs: 4g
85% fat, 6% protein, 9% carbs

INGREDIENT TIP: Tahini is ground sesame seeds. You'll find it either in the refrigerated section near the dairy products in health food stores or in shelf-stable jars in the ethnic foods section of the grocery store.

Pesto

VEGETARIAN • 30 MINUTES OR LESS

KETO
QUOTIENT

1 2 ③

Pesto adds so much flavor to sauces, vegetables, and meats. It's a great way to use leftover fresh basil if you purchased a large bunch for another recipe. If you don't have pine nuts, feel free to swap them for another nut, such as pecans or pistachios.

2 cups fresh basil leaves

¼ teaspoon sea salt

1 garlic clove

½ cup extra-virgin olive oil

¼ cup ground pine nuts

¼ cup grated Parmesan cheese

1. In a blender, blend the basil, salt, garlic, and olive oil until mostly smooth.

2. Stir in the pine nuts and Parmesan cheese. Serve immediately or store in a covered container in the refrigerator for up to two days.

PER SERVING (2 tablespoons) Calories: 158; Fat: 17g; Protein: 2g; Total Carbs: 1g; Fiber: 1g; Net Carbs: 0g; 97% fat, 2% protein, 1% carbs

PREP TIP: Pour this pesto into an ice cube tray and freeze so you can pop out a cube whenever you need it for a recipe.

Chicken Bone Broth

KETO QUOTIENT
① 2 3

Yields 2 quarts / Prep time: 5 minutes / Cook time: 4 hours

DAIRY FREE • NUT FREE

Bone broth is a good source of electrolytes, which are often in short supply on low-carb diets as your body sheds excess water weight. You can use it in soups, stews, and sauces. Alternatively, it makes a delicious beverage for sipping between meals.

1 pound chicken bones,
    preferably roasted
1 tablespoon apple cider vinegar

1 teaspoon sea salt
4 quarts cold water

1. Place the chicken bones, vinegar, and salt in a large pot. Cover with the water and bring to a simmer over medium heat. Reduce the heat to medium-low and simmer for 4 hours, or until reduced to about 2 quarts.

2. Allow the stock to cool completely before storing in a covered container in the refrigerator for up to 1 week or in the freezer for up to 3 months.

PER SERVING (1 cup) Calories: 45; Fat: 1g; Protein: 9g; Total Carbs: 0g; Fiber: 0g; Net Carbs: 0g
20% fat, 80% protein, 0% carbs

PREP TIP: I like to use leftover chicken bones from a whole roasted chicken. Alternatively, toss the bones onto a baking sheet and coat with 1 tablespoon of oil. Roast at 400°F for 20 minutes, or until browned.

Beef Bone Broth

Yields 2 quarts / Prep time: 4 minutes / Cook time: 4 hours 40 minutes

DAIRY FREE • NUT FREE

Beef bone broth is loaded with flavor and becomes even more concentrated as you cook it down. In fact, you can continue cooking until the bone broth is reduced to a mere two cups of liquid for a decadent demi-glace.

1 pound beef bones

1 tablespoon apple cider vinegar

1 teaspoon sea salt

4 quarts water

1. Preheat the oven to 400°F. Spread the beef bones out onto a rimmed baking sheet. Roast uncovered for 40 minutes, or until browned.

2. Transfer the beef bones to a large pot. Pour the oil from the roasting pan and use a fat separator to discard the fat. Transfer the remaining bits, called the fond, to the pot.

3. Add the vinegar, salt, and water to the pot and bring to a gentle simmer. Cook partially covered for 4 hours, skimming fat off the surface as it rises.

4. Allow the stock to cool completely before storing in a covered container in the refrigerator for up to 1 week or in the freezer for up to 3 months.

PER SERVING Calories: 45; Fat: 1g; Protein: 9g; Total Carbs: 0g; Fiber: 0g; Net Carbs: 0g
20% fat, 80% protein, 0% carbs

INGREDIENT TIP: Don't skip the step of roasting the bones; otherwise, the broth will have a slightly metallic taste.

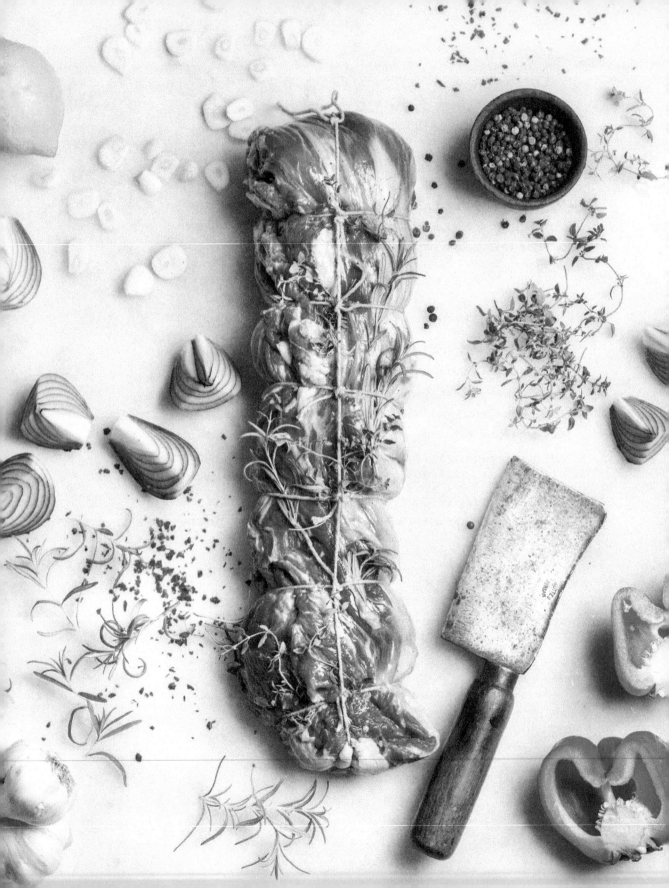

Measurement Conversions

Volume Equivalents (Dry)

US Standard	Metric (approximate)
⅛ teaspoon	0.5 mL
¼ teaspoon	1 mL
½ teaspoon	2 mL
¾ teaspoon	4 mL
1 teaspoon	5 mL
1 tablespoon	15 mL
¼ cup	59 mL
⅓ cup	79 mL
½ cup	118 mL
⅔ cup	156 mL
¾ cup	177 mL
1 cup	235 mL
2 cups or 1 pint	475 mL
3 cups	700 mL
4 cups or 1 quart	1 L
½ gallon	2 L
1 gallon	4 L

Volume Equivalents (Liquid)

US Standard	US Standard (ounces)	Metric (approximate)
2 tablespoons	1 fl. oz.	30 mL
¼ cup	2 fl. oz.	60 mL
½ cup	4 fl. oz.	120 mL
1 cup	8 fl. oz.	240 mL
1½ cups	12 fl. oz.	355 mL
2 cups or 1 pint	16 fl. oz.	475 mL
4 cups or 1 quart	32 fl. oz.	1 L
1 gallon	128 fl. oz.	4 L

Oven Temperatures

Fahrenheit (F)	Celsius (C) (approximate)
250°F	120°C
300°F	150°C
325°F	165°C
350°F	180°C
375°F	190°C
400°F	200°C
425°F	220°C
450°F	230°C

Weight Equivalents

US Standard	Metric (approximate)
½ ounce	15 g
1 ounce	30 g
2 ounces	60 g
4 ounces	115 g
8 ounces	225 g
12 ounces	340 g
16 ounces or 1 pound	455 g

APPENDIX B
The Dirty Dozen and the Clean Fifteen

A nonprofit and environmental watchdog organization called Environmental Working Group (EWG) looks at data supplied by the US Department of Agriculture (USDA) and the Food and Drug Administration (FDA) about pesticide residues and compiles a list each year of the best and worst pesticide loads found in commercial crops. You can refer to the Dirty Dozen list to know which fruits and vegetables you should always buy organic. The Clean Fifteen list lets you know which produce is considered safe enough when grown conventionally to allow you to skip the organics. This does not mean that the Clean Fifteen produce is pesticide-free, though, so wash these fruits and vegetables thoroughly.

These lists change every year, so make sure you look up the most recent before you fill your shopping cart. You'll find the most recent lists as well as a guide to pesticides in produce at EWG.org/FoodNews.

2017 Dirty Dozen		2017 Clean Fifteen	
Apples	Strawberries	Asparagus	Onions
Celery	Sweet bell peppers	Avocados	Papayas
Cherry tomatoes	*In addition to the Dirty Dozen, the EWG added two foods contaminated with highly toxic organophosphate insecticides:*	Cabbage	Pineapples
Cucumbers		Cantaloupe	Sweet corn
Grapes		Cauliflower	Sweet peas (frozen)
Nectarines		Eggplant	
Peaches	*Hot peppers*	Grapefruit	Sweet potatoes
Potatoes	Kale/Collard greens	Kiwis	
Snap peas		Mangoes	
Spinach			

References

De Luis, D., J.C. Domingo, O. Izaolo, F.F. Casanueva, D. Bellido, and I. Sajoux. "Effect of DHA Supplementation in a Very Low-Calorie Ketogenic Diet in the Treatment of Obesity: A Randomized Clinical Trial." *Endocrine* 54, no. 1 (October 2016): 111–122. doi:10.1007/s12020-016-0964-z

Ervin, R. Bethene, PhD, RD, and Cynthia L. Ogden, PhD, MRP. "Consumption of Added Sugars Among US Adults, 2005–2010." National Center for Health Statistics. Accessed March 9, 2017. www.cdc.gov/nchs/data/databriefs/db122.pdf

Flynn, M.M., and S.E. Reinert. "Comparing an Olive Oil-Enriched Diet to a Standard Lower-Fat Diet for Weight Loss in Breast Cancer Survivors: A Pilot Study." *Journal of Women's Health* 19, no. 6 (June 2010): 1155-61. doi: 10.1089/jwh.2009.1759

Gomez-Arbelaez, D., D. Bellido, A.I. Castro, L. Ordoñez-Mayan, J. Carreira, C. Galban, M.A. Martinez-Olmos, A.B. Crujeiras, I. Sajoux, F.F. Casanueva. "Body Composition Changes After Very-Low-Calorie Ketogenic Diet in Obesity Evaluated by Three Standardized Methods." *Journal of Clinical Endocrinology and Metabolism* 102, no. 2 (February 2017): 488–498. doi: 10.1210/jc.2016-2385

Haddad, E., et al., "A Randomized 3 x 3 Crossover Study to Evaluate the Effect of Hass Avocado Intake on Post-Ingestive Satiety, Glucose and Insulin Levels, and Subsequent Energy Intake in Overweight Adults." *Nutrition Journal* 12, no. 155 (November 2013). doi: 10.1186/1475-2891-12-155

Hendon, Louise. "What Are the Optimal Ketone Levels for a Ketogenic Diet?" *Paleo Magazine*. Accessed April 6, 2017. https://paleomagazine.com/optimal-ketone-levels-for-ketogenic-diet#how-to-interpret-ketone-levels

Saslow, L.R., A.E. Mason, S. Kim, V. Goldman, R. Ploutz-Snyder, H. Bayandorian, J. Daubenmier, F.M. Hecht, and J.T. Moskowitz. "An Online Intervention Comparing a Very Low-Carbohydrate Ketogenic Diet and Lifestyle Recommendations Versus a Plate Method Diet in Overweight Individuals With Type 2 Diabetes: A Randomized Controlled Trial." *J Med Internet Res* 19, no. 2 (February 2017): e36. doi: 10.2196/jmir.5806

Taubes, Gary. *Why We Get Fat: And What to Do About It*. New York City, NY: Anchor Books, 2011.

Urbain, P., and H. Bertz. "Monitoring for Compliance with a Ketogenic Diet: What Is the Best Time of Day to Test for Urinary Ketosis?" *Nutr Metab* (Lond) 13, no. 77 (November 2016). doi:10.1186/s12986-016-0136-4

WebMD. "What is Ketosis?" Type 1 Diabetes Guide, WebMD. Accessed April 6, 2017. www.webmd.com/diabetes/type-1-diabetes-guide/what-is-ketosis#1

Zelman, Kathleen M., MPH, RD, LD. "It's Full of Fat and Helps You Lose Weight." Diet and Weight Management, WebMD. Accessed April 6, 2017. www.webmd.com/diet/features/its-full-fat-and-helps-you-lose-weight#1

Recipe Index

Index

About the Author

PAMELA ELLGEN is a private chef who works with weight-loss clients to help them achieve their goals one meal at a time. She is the author of more than a dozen books on fitness, nutrition, and cooking, including *The Microbiome Cookbook, Cast Iron Paleo*, and *The Gluten-Free Cookbook for Families.* She lives in Santa Barbara, California, with her husband and two sons. When she's not in the kitchen, you can find her surfing or exploring the local farmers' market.